Sex Positions

KAMA SUTRA & TANTRIC SEX

---
2 BOOKS IN 1

Transform Your Sexual Life. Awake the ultimate pleasure with illustrated sex positions, spicy ideas, and sex games

SAMANTHA MANDALA

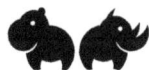

IPPOCERONTE
publishing

KAMA SUTRA
Sex Guide for Couples

&

TANTRIC SEX
Guide for Couples

SAMANTHA MANDALA

CONTENTS

KAMA SUTRA
Sex Guide for Couples

The Ultimate Fully Illustrated Book for Beginners and Advanced to Master Sex Positions, Discover New Kinky Ideas with Your Partner and Transform Your Sex Life.

SAMANTHA MANDALA

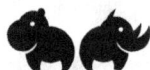

IPPOCERONTE
publishing

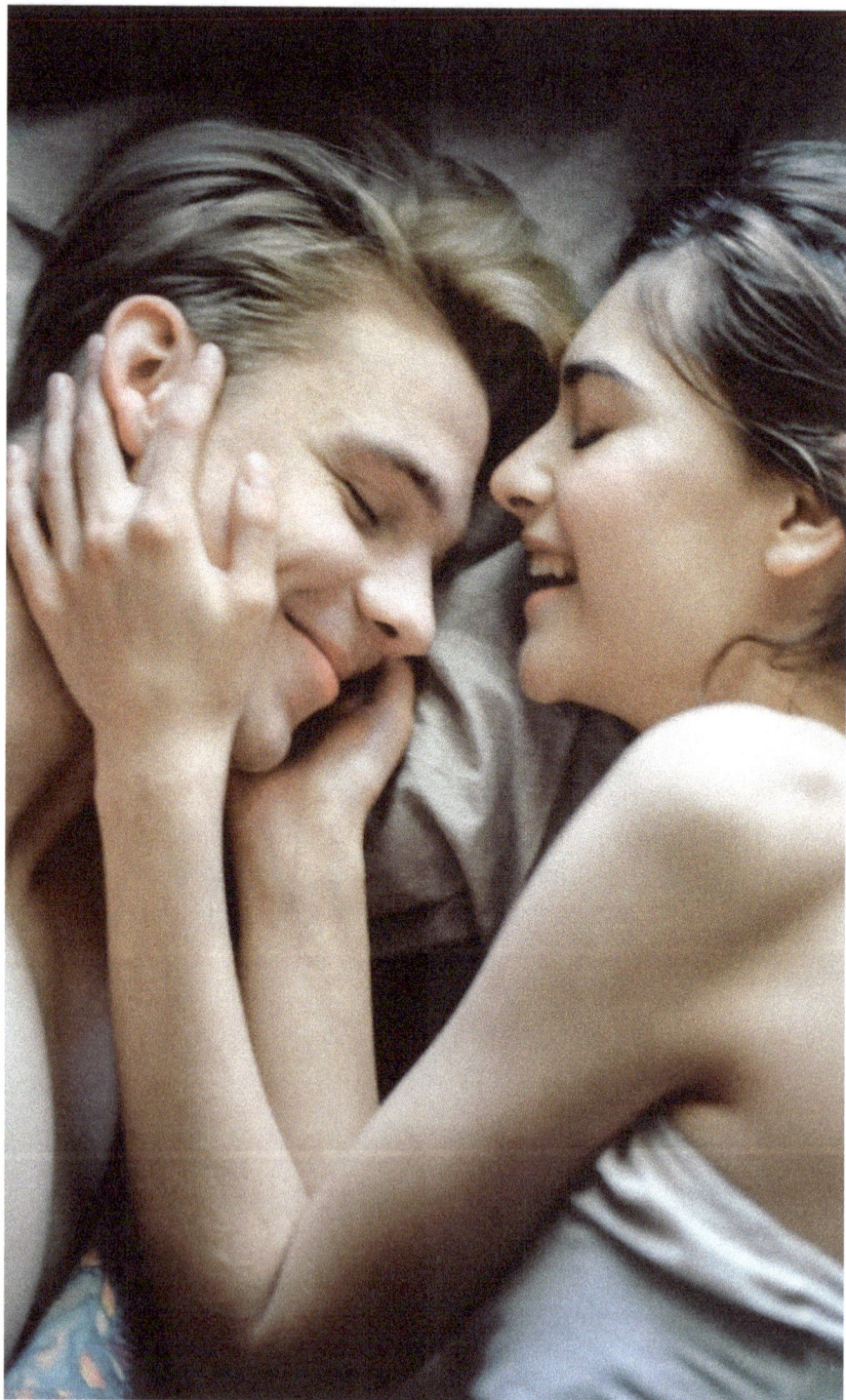

Introduction

In Sanskrit, the Kama Sutra - or "love scripture" - is one of the most known texts on love and sexuality from ancient India. In this opera, we will explore some aspects covered in the original text and see how they are relevant to modern relationships. This book is aimed at experienced couples and individuals who are going to begin a relationship. It is for the individuals who do not just want to stop at the sexual act, but they want to improve their relationship in every aspect. Furthermore, particularly for those for whom love and trust are equivalent words, who are prepared not exclusively to take yet, in addition, to give something as a tradeoff. This book will help you build a stronger relationship, avoid the most common mistakes, and break down the obstacles that prevent you from achieving pleasure.

What is more, this isn't unexpected, because we are on the whole individuals of Western culture. In the interim, Eastern demeanor to erotic love is drastically not quite the same as the sexual culture of the West. It might not come as a surprise, but the concept of sensuality in Eastern culture is vastly different from what can be found in Western cultures. In Hinduism, the body and otherworldly life, sexuality, and purity were viewed as a single entity. All the old-fashioned oriental compositions on the craft of love were committed to the mystical side of sex, and the Kama Sutra is maybe perhaps the most popular.

Even today, the Kama Sutra continues to help countless couples, assisting them with figuring out how to control their mind, body, feelings, and sexual arousal, permitting them to discover opportunity and congruity in personal life.

In this book, I will do my best to explain the core of the Kama Sutra and all its various facets. We will discuss areas like foreplay, flirting, sensual fantasies, fetishes, and everything that can be used to improve the relationship with your partner and keep the spark alive. By perusing this book, you will locate a whole armory of all sexual positions introduced in the Kama Sutra.

You will become more familiar with magical sexual ceremonies, strategies for postponing orgasm, oral sex, and different parts of sexuality. I will do my best to pass on the information contained in the Kama Sutra, in a basic and clear language, in a structure wholly adjusted to the view of the individual of our day.

Bit by bit, this book inspects all the normal strides of sexual intercourse between partners - from the principal kisses and lovemaking to the mysteries of a fantastic orgasm. The variety of procedures and techniques contained in this book will not permit your relationship to transform into a daily schedule. The other way around, you can continually find an ever-increasing number of new vibes that have never been capable.

It will not be too difficult even to consider dominating these stunts, and the result will surpass every one of your assumptions. Thus, if you need to uncover your sexual potential and become an eager, incredibly creative lover, at that point, this book is the thing that you need!

CHAPTER 1

Your First Steps into Kama Sutra

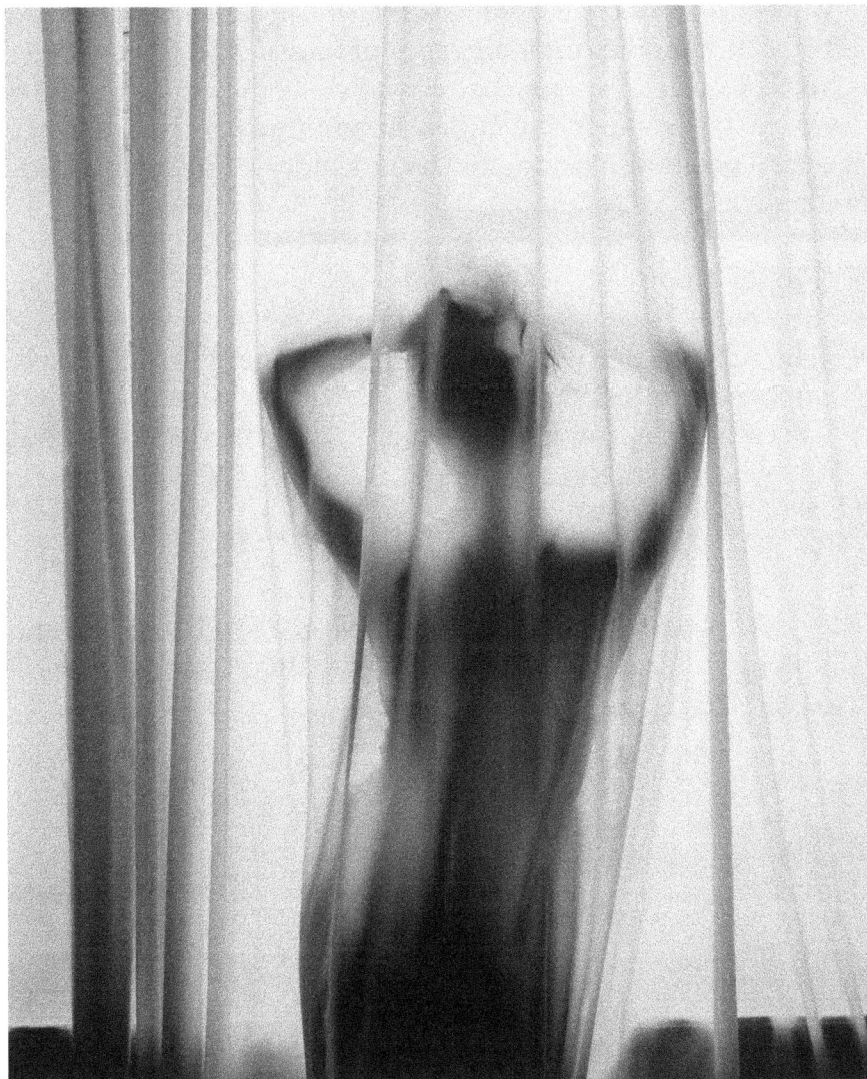

1.1 THE MEANING

The Kama Sutra is an ancient Indian book that reviews human sexual conduct. It is viewed as vital work in Sanskrit writing, which has love, desire, happiness, energy, and sensuality, just as sexuality in the strict sense. The Kama Sutra was composed around the second century by Vatsyayana, and the genuine title of the book is Vatsyayana Kama Sutra, or "Maxims on the love of Vatsyayana." It is believed that some parts of the Kama Sutra have been added posthumously. For instance, the original text did not contain the different types of kisses. These techniques have been added by a translator who wished to make the book more useful for modern couples. In addition to a varied range of sexual positions, the original text includes many other topics, among which we can find:

- Proper grooming and self-care
- Etiquette, including appropriate post-coital conversation
- The practice of the arts, ranging from poetry to cooking to mixing perfumes
- Discretion in conducting affairs, particularly adulterous ones
- Homosexual desire
- Female sexuality

The Kama is part of the four permissible goals of Hindu life and commonly refers to pleasure. In the following chapter, we will see each of these goals in more detail.

1.2 PURUSHARTHAS: THE FOUR MAIN GOALS OF LIFE

According to ancient Indian philosophy, every human has four good goals, called *Purushartha*. They are the pillars that define a satisfying, meaningful life. Being able to live according to these ideals is not easy but highly satisfying.

Dharma: This is the desire to live righteously and do good deeds. For Hindu, *Dharma* includes moral rights, religious duties, and duties of each individual. It is essential to understand your ethical obligations and follow them; otherwise, you will have many regrets and end up in an unpleasant situation where you always look over your shoulder for karma coming to get you.

Artha: *Artha* has many meanings; it can be translated as "wealth," "money," "resources," or "means of life." But here, it refers specifically to material wealth or prosperity. It does not refer to the mindless accumulation of money; instead, it means working hard to achieve financial stability and economic prosperity.

Kama: the *Kama* signifies passions, emotions, desire for sensual pleasure. The Kama can be defined as *"love without violating Dharma"* (your moral responsibilities). It also includes worldly pleasures such as fine food and leisure activities like reading or watching movies.

Moksha: *Moksha* is the desire to let go of all worldly desires and find true enlightenment. In some interpretations connotes freedom from the cycle of death and rebirth, while others signify self-knowledge, self-realization, and liberation in this life. Some people are content to have these three first, but you should stand firm in your beliefs and make whatever sacrifices are necessary to achieve the fourth!

1.3 HISTORY OF KAMA SUTRA

The Kama Sutra is an ancient Indian Sanskrit text on sensuality, the specific date that the Kama Sutra was composed is not known. Yet, gauges place it anyplace between 400 BCE and 300 CE. What we do know, notwithstanding, is that it was authoritatively accumulated and transformed into the book that we know today in the second century. However, this does not mean that the book has not gone through updates from that point forward. A few researchers accept that the adaptation we have is entirely connected to the third century, as a portion of the references all through would not have been relevant to the second century. With the content being so old, dating the manuscript is practically impossible. The opera is attributed to *Vatsyayana*, an ancient Indian philosopher that lived in India (Pataliputra) during the second CE.

Despite the common conception that it is a book containing mainly sexual positions, the Kama Sutra is much more than this. It is written as a guide to the art of living well, understanding the nature of love, finding a life partner, or keeping the flame of passion alight.

It is essential to realize that **Kama Sutra never stops evolving**. What was relevant a few centuries ago might be less important now, but the core principles of the Kama Sutra are always current. After this brief introduction to Kama Sutra, we will dive directly into the middle of the action. According to the original text, the act of lovemaking is divided into four steps, all equally important:

- Preparation
- Foreplay
- Sexual Congress
- Afterplay

Each of these steps will be deepened in the course of this book and, if necessary, enriched with a more modern vision.

~ CHAPTER 2 ~
The First Stage of Lovemaking - Preparation

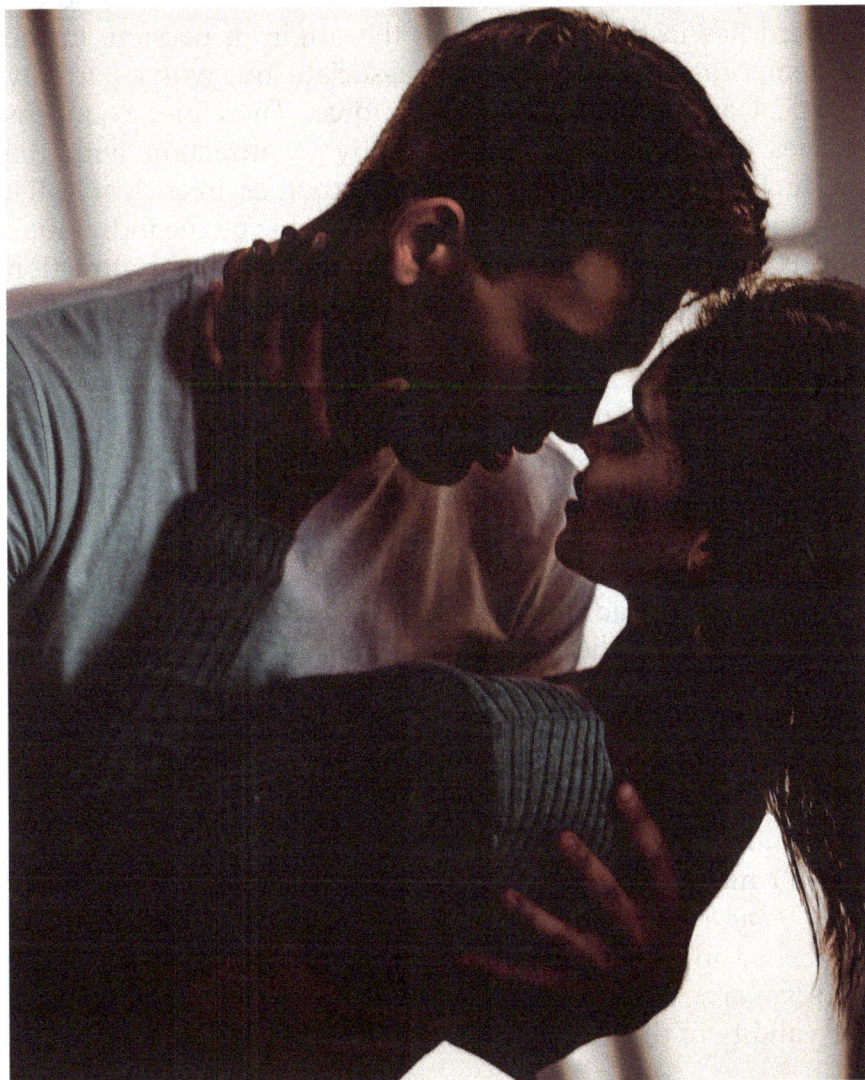

2.1 SEDUCTION AND RESPECT

Even if it does not include new exotic sexual positions, the preparation stage is crucial for the Kama Sutra. And in the original text, ample space is devoted to this topic. An essential part of the Kama Sutra is dedicated to the *art of seduction* and its many facets.

One of the main differences between the ancient world and the modern lies in the beliefs about the origin of passion. In the contemporary world, we tend to associate love with a partially mystical and partially biological force. Therefore, countless studies on the subject aim to motivate attraction with the production of certain substances in our bodies. In ancient India, it was believed that passion was controllable by the individual, that it was possible to create and maintain sexual attraction through various erotic practices. The ancient Indians did not understand the chemical reactions in our bodies and believed that passion was a force subject to a well-trained mind. The original version of the Kama Sutra was full of seduction advice. Some might sound strange nowadays, while others might be helpful if interpreted in a modern key.

Play hard to get

The original text advises women to push men away (at first), especially during the first dates; women should try to reduce physical contact and make themselves desired as much as possible. Yes, we all know this story. But, I think, a couple of thousand years ago, this advice might not have been so obvious! The text also contains a strategy for men, which consists of frequently yawning and touching their mustache. Ok, this doesn't make much sense. However, we must bear in mind that *"Play hard to get,"* according to science, works. A study published in *"Psychological sciences"* entitled *"He loves me, He loves me not ...: uncertainty can increase romantic attraction"* proved the validity of the theory through a social experiment.

The researchers showed to several women Facebook profiles of possible partners. First, a group of women was told that the man found them extremely attractive and would like to have a first date. Then, the second group of women was told that the potential partner found them attractive enough, while the last group of women was told that the partner was unsure of his feelings towards them.Guess which men were found sexier by women? Primarily those belonging to the last group, men uncertain of their feelings!

Seduction is about the ritual
In the original version of the Kama Sutra, various courtship rituals were described, which today would no longer make much sense. Nothing was left to chance, and everything was carefully orchestrated to achieve the maximum chance of success. I do not think we would have anything to learn from these rituals if taken literally. At least, I do not see how it would help me in real life to tickle my partner's feet with lotus flowers. However, we can learn as a lesson to **regularly allocate enough time to spend with the person we love**. Create your ritual, choose a night of the week, and make it your special evening. Despite all the problems and stress you may have, make room for one night a week and spend it with your partner!

Respect your partner
I have to be honest with you; the Kama Sutra is full of patriarchal nonsense. However, we must never forget that the text was written in ancient times and from a completely different culture. Despite this, the Kama Sutra contains some pearls of wisdom.
For example, the book advises wives not to use harsh words with their husbands in public and deal with them privately. Furthermore, a wife should never divulge the secrets her husband confides to him. These, although obvious, are valuable pieces of advice that nowadays obviously apply to both genders. It is vital to building a relationship based on trust and collaboration with your partner so you can create a protected space in which to be yourself.

2.2 LEAVE THE REST OF THE WORLD OUTSIDE

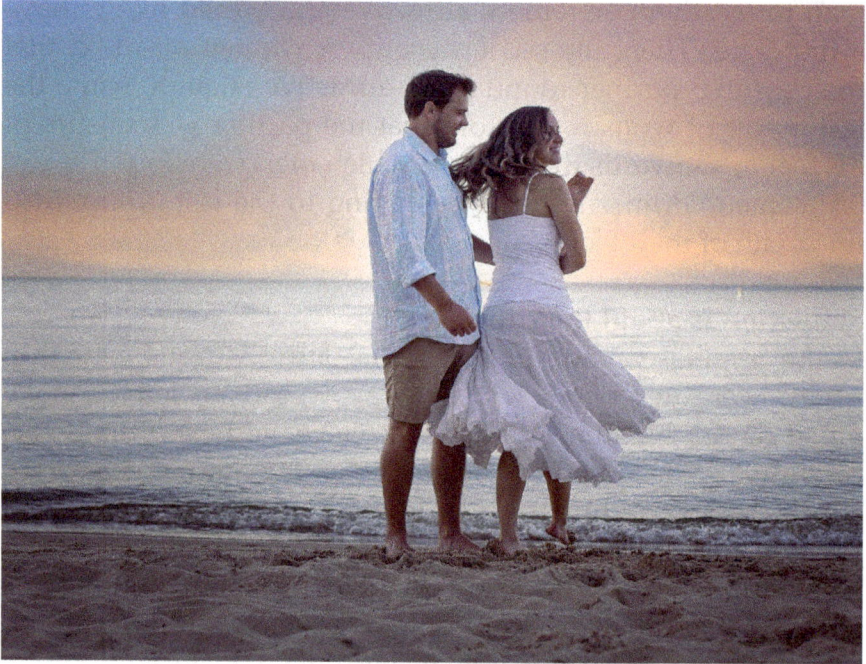

Kama sutra is not for everyday sex; it requires time and patience. Kama sutra can help to forget about day-to-day problems if both partners have the will to invest time and effort in achieving the pleasure together. It is essential to understand that Kama Sutra requires a particular effort, and it is crucial to allocate a reasonable amount of time to be spent with the partner. The end goal is not exclusively having sex but to get to know your partner intimately.

You want to build a strong relationship based on collaboration, trust, and mutual respect.

The first and more important rule is: **Leave the rest of the world outside.**

Decide for how much time you want to commit and make an effort to leave all the day's problems behind. Then, you must reach the awareness that for a few hours, it will be just you and your partner.

Leave all distractions, problems, chores, and appointments outside; it is just the two of you.

2.3 SETTING THE SCENE

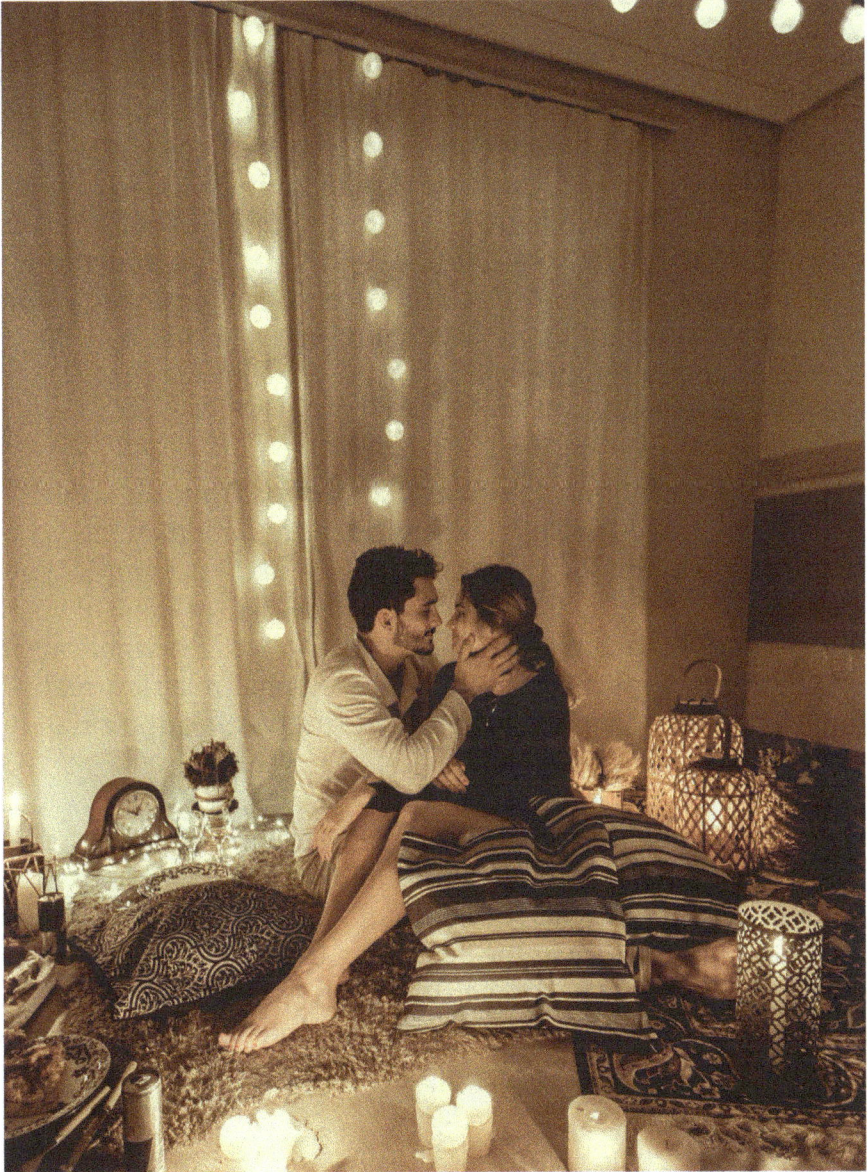

A quiet evening at home might be just the ticket to a romantic interlude, or you might want to rent a room in a luxurious hotel. Hundreds of ideas can help to set the right mood. Just keep in mind the relationship that you have built with your partner so far and what they like. In some cases, especially at the beginning of your relationship, you might want to keep it simple.

Here are some ideas that I hope can give you inspiration for your spicy evenings.

Get the right food: One of the best ways to enhance the mood is to make sure the room is stocked with the necessities. I personally love an excellent Champagne, but any other beverage that you both like will do the job. Strawberries or other fruit already sliced are always appreciated and can be used during the foreplay as well. Also, consider buying some chocolate and do not forget water and ice cubes. You may want to rehydrate during the evening or use the ice to play with hot and cold sensations!

Send your partner an invite and an outfit: You can surprise your partner by sending them a written invitation, along with a box that contains a fantastic outfit to wear. For example, you could pick something that your partner will like or think of your most favorite fantasy vixen and go with that. The right outfit could be the perfect opportunity to do some roleplay, realize your fantasies or simply be sure your partner is appropriately dressed for an elegant evening.

Candles dimmable lights: With a few minor additions, it is easy to transform your house into the perfect background for sensual adventures with your partner. You can set some candles on the dinner table, near the bed, or on the edge of the bathtub. Changing the lights is a powerful way to set the scene; shadows and lights are the perfect way to make more appealing the old bed and ignite passion.

Sounds: Music can help to create the right atmosphere. Pick something that you both like, or go for less invasive instrumental music. You might also consider non-music soundtracks like various sounds of nature: waves, birds, wind, etc. If your house is a bit noisy or you are not alone, you could use a white noise machine to block outside noise and cover bedroom noise.

Scents: Perfumes and scented powders are lovely (if you do not exceed with them). I love to burn some incense; sandalwood, ylang-ylang, and jasmine can stimulate sexual appetite and increase sexual attraction. If this is not your cup of tea, you could lightly scent your linens instead. Also, scented candles and air fresheners are a good alternative.

Take a bath together: Nothing is better than taking a bath together to release the tension. Sounds, smells, candles, and dimmable lights can be used in various combinations to wash away all the stress and awake your senses. It is an extraordinary chance to purify your day out and start new with your accomplice. In the Kama Sutra, it is expressed that the two accomplices ought to be newly purified after going into the pleasure room. This is to ensure that you are perfect and that your body is attractive to your accomplice.

2.4 TWELVE EMBRACES

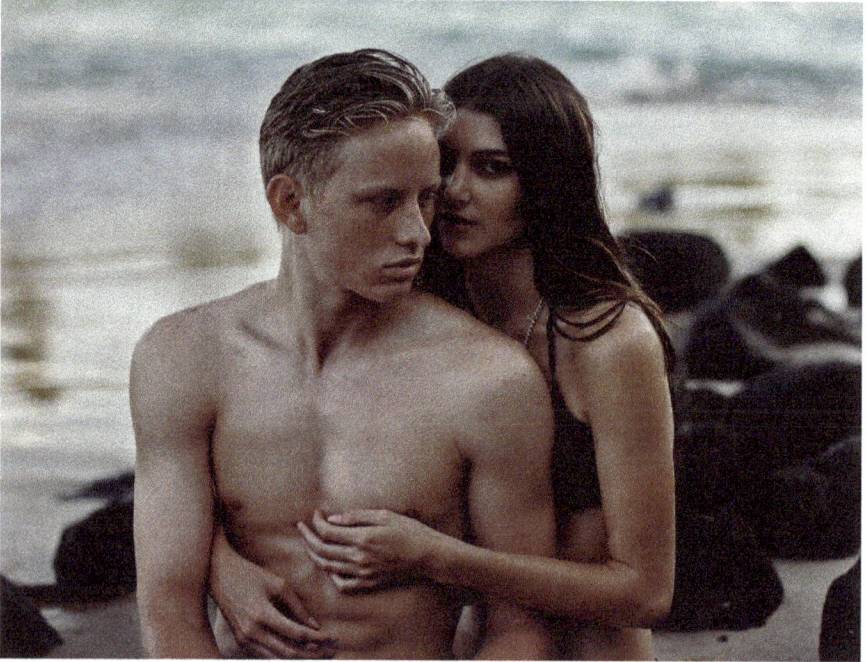

In the original book, various types of embraces are described. They can be used during all the stages of lovemaking, and there is one for every different situation.

Embracing can be an easy route to start some foreplay or just a way to show affection to your partner. For couples who are obscure to each other, embracing is an extraordinary method to eliminate the distance between them. However, a couple who knows about each other may move toward embracing with a drive.

Some of these hugs will seem obvious and not particularly creative, but I have chosen to report them in this book for completeness. We must keep in mind that the original text was written at a time when it was not easy to deal openly with any sexual subject matter. For this reason, even an obvious list of hugs was crucial educational material.

Touching embrace

According to the original Kama Sutra: *"When a man under some pretext or other goes in front of or alongside a woman and touches her body with his own, it is called the touching embrace."*

This embrace is an unexpected soft touch. It is a subtle display of affection, reminding your partner that you are still there and of what is to come. Soft unforeseen touches throughout the day will do wonders in preparing your partner for the night of love ahead.

Piercing embrace

In this embrace, the woman bends a bit to press her breasts against her man's body to tease him. This will ignite the flames of desire between them, which in turn makes the man reach for her breasts.

Rubbing embrace

A rubbing embrace is a public act that shows both love and desire. According to the Kama Sutra: *"When two lovers are strolling together, either in the dark, or in a place of public resort, or a lonely place, and rub their bodies against each other, it is called a rubbing embrace."*

Pressing embrace

"When on the occasion of walking together a lover presses the other's body forcibly against a wall or pillar, it is called a pressing embrace." This, more than a single embrace, is a variation of the other embraces. It is perfect during pre-sexual foreplay; it helps ignite passion and raise the temperature.

Twining of a creeper (Jataveshtotaka)

According to Kama Sutra: *"When a woman, clinging to a man as a creeper twines around a tree, bends his head down to hers with the desire of kissing him and slightly makes the sound of sut sut, embraces him, and looks lovingly toward him, it is called an embrace like the twining of a creeper."*

It might be challenging to know what the sound of "*sut sut*" sounds like; what is essential with this embrace is understanding that it would just occur in private. This embrace is a very personal one and is a display of physical affection given by the woman.

Climbing a tree (Vrikshadhirudhaka)
The woman embraces her lover by placing one hand around his shoulder, reaching for the back with the other, while placing one of her feet on his thighs. Then she set the other foot on her lover's foot, just as if she were about to climb a tree and all her moves express her desire to acquire a kiss from her sexual partner.

Milk and water embrace (Kshiraniraka)
This embrace can be interpreted as dry sex in modern terms. According to Kama Sutra:

"When a man and a woman are very much in love with each other, and, not thinking of any pain or hurt, embrace each other as if they were entering into each other's bodies either while the woman is sitting on the lap of the man, or in front of him, or on a bed, then it is called an embrace like a mixture of milk and water."

The Kshiraniraka embrace is close to having sex, but with the clothes on. It is used to express passion and has a vast erotic charge. There is only a thin barrier of cloth to stop the couple from having actual sex.

The mixture of sesamum seed with rice (Tila-Tandulaka)
During this embrace, you lie in bed, either scooping or being scooped by the other. That is close to what this kind of embrace is all about. Whether you lie down face to face with each other or facing your back to your partner, you both should be lying next to each other with your arms and legs entwining each other.

Embrace of the Jaghana
According to the Kama Sutra:

"When a man presses the jaghana of a woman's body against his own and mounts upon her to practice scratching with the nail or finger, biting, striking or kissing, the hair of the woman being loose and flowing, it is called the embrace of the jaghana."

Jaghana is the area between the navel and the thighs. This embrace mixes pain and pleasure and can be an extremely sensual and erotic experience. We will see later in this book, in more detail, the arts of scratching and biting and how these can stimulate sexual arousal.

Embrace of the thighs
This is a very simple embrace that doesn't require a long description; it is when the lovers squeeze each other's thighs with theirs.

Embrace of the breasts
This is the kind of embrace that would occur later during foreplay. According to Kama Sutra, *"When a man places his breast between the breasts of a woman and presses her with it, it is called the embrace of the breasts."*

Embrace of the forehead
According to Kama Sutra: *"When either of the lovers touches the mouth, the eyes, and the forehead of the other with his or her own, it is called the embrace of the forehead."* This embrace is a very personal one, with the faces of the two lovers coming into contact. Nevertheless, it is a gentle gesture of affection and suitable for any stage of lovemaking.

~ CHAPTER 3 ~

The Second Stage of Lovemaking - Foreplay

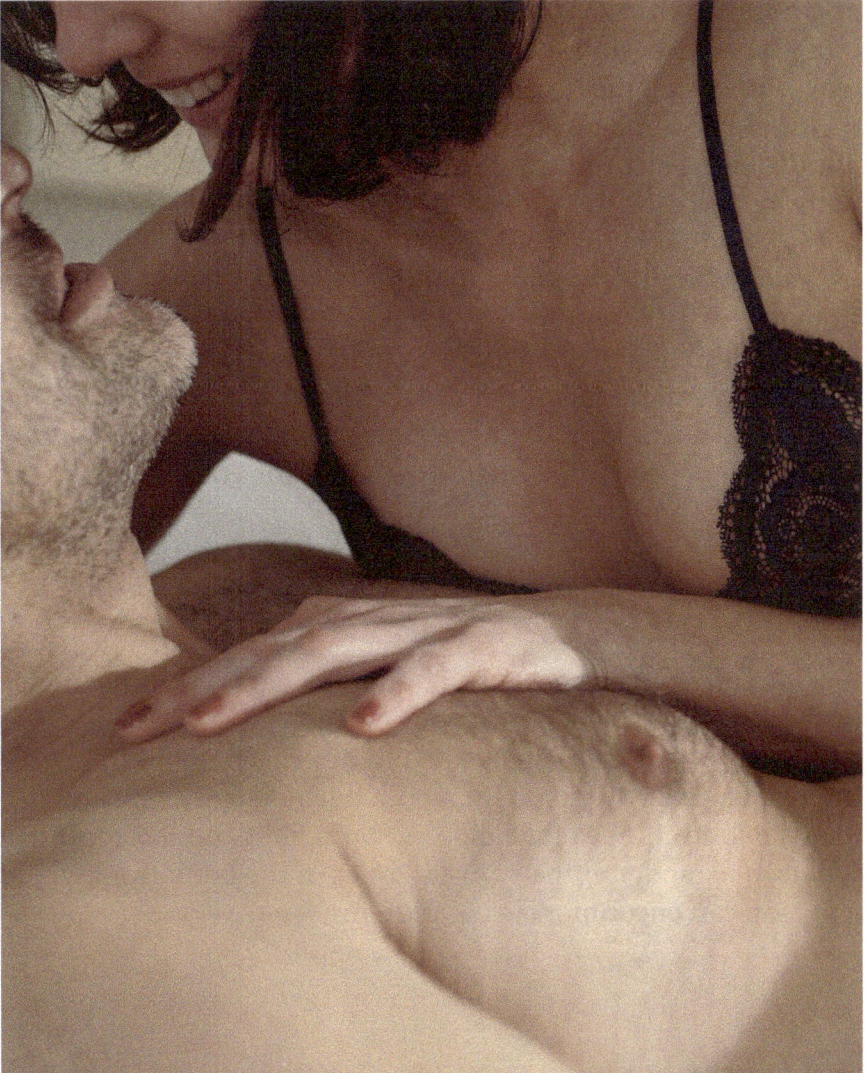

The foreplay is a set of emotionally and physically intimate acts between two or more people meant to create sexual arousal and desire for sexual activity. The foreplay is what warms the environment and leads to sex. Its primary purpose is to generate excitement and prepare the two partners to make love.

We are all captivated by the sex scenes of the films, by the garments that fly conspicuously all around, and by the bodies that rapidly end up between the sheets. In the collective imagination, this is cool and sometimes might happen, but in most cases, everything starts before, in a moderate and fragile way, without all the display. When foreplay was worked out in the original Kama Sutra, there was a reference to the servants who might help the man arrange the room before meeting with his lady. In the present society, large numbers of us do not have workers that we can depend on to do these things for us. Consequently, the content of this chapter has been adjusted from the way it was originally written. It is now more connected with modern society than to the Indian culture of a few centuries ago. This chapter will mix some techniques that were part of the original Kama Sutra with more modern approaches. Hopefully, you will find here some interesting ideas for your foreplay.

3.1 EROGENOUS ZONES

A wide range of areas can be stimulated from multiple angles during the foreplay to excite your partner.
Knowing where these areas are and approaching them is very important; this will ensure that both partners are ready and full of desire once the sexual congress starts.First and foremost, we will take a gander at the various zones of the body from which a person can encounter sexual pleasure.

Bottoms of feet

Feet have been the object of desire for a century. Some people love them, and some people hate them. Regardless of whether you are a foot lover or not, it is essential to know that feet have many nerve endings and pressure points; stimulating this often-neglected area with a massage or a soft touch can lead to pleasurable sensations.

Armpits

Inner arms and armpits are susceptible areas where many people are touchy. You can use a soft touch along this area to stimulate the nerves and ignite the flame. If you feel kinky, why do not play with a feather and torment your partner? Based on their body's response, you can mix tickling and sexual arousal.

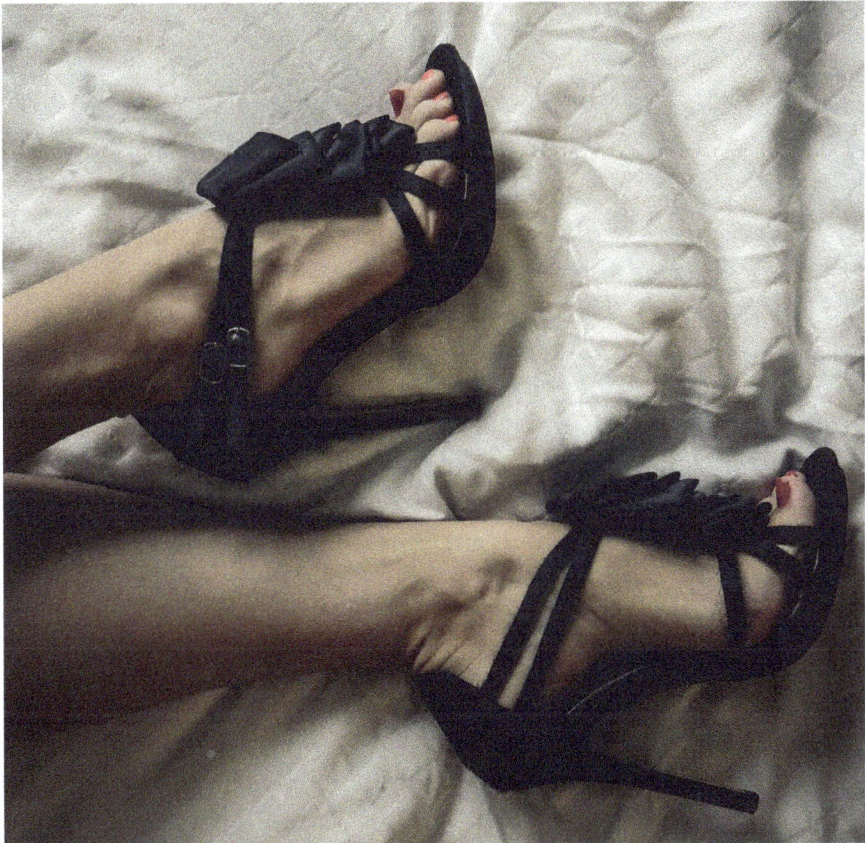

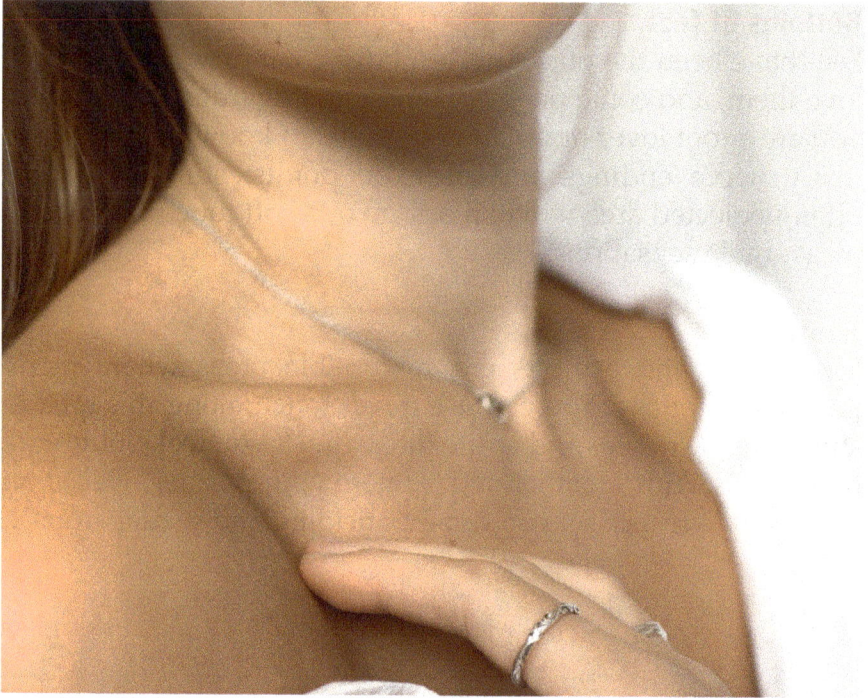

Neck

The neck is one of the most popular and sensitive erogenous zones, from the nape at the back of the neck to the sides below the jawline. Many people enjoy stimulation along the neck with a light touch or kissing.

Inner thighs

The inner thighs are incredibly close to genital areas and particularly sensitive. You can try a light touch while moving towards the genitals; your partner will love it!

Behind the knee

This area might come as a surprise but behind the knee is another sensitive, nerve-rich area of the body. In most cases, this area is ignored, but trust me, paying particular attention to it during a full-body massage can elicit arousal.

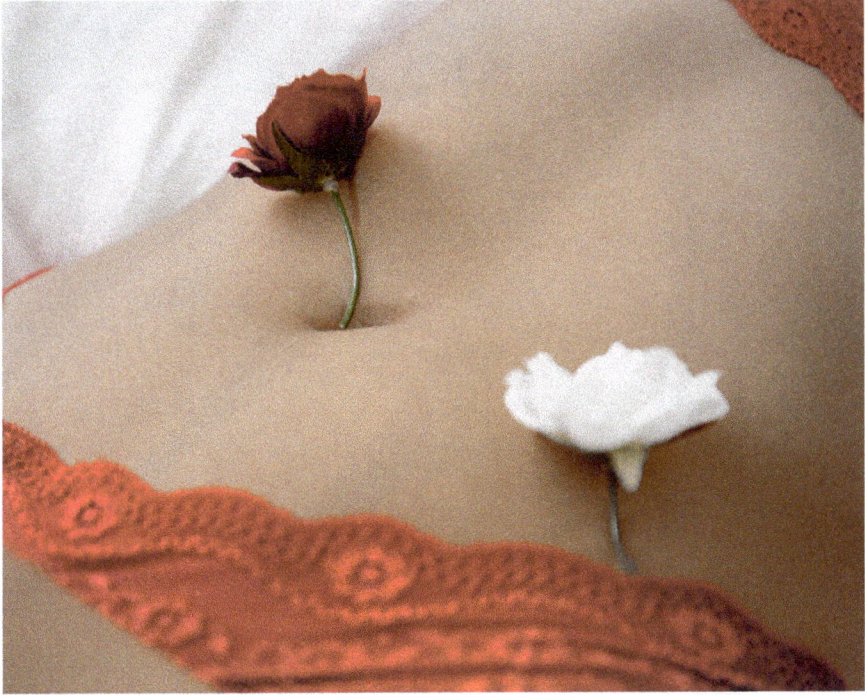

Lower stomach and belly button

The lower abdomen and belly button are incredibly sensitive areas, and they have the advantage of being near the genital region. A light touch near these areas can easily lead to sexual arousal.

Ears

The ears are full of nerves and sensory receptors, and they are one of the most sensitive erogenous zones in the human body. From the tip to the lob, there is not a single spot that will not elicit arousal.

You can play with them in various ways; light nibbles or kisses are a good ice breaker, and, depending on what your partner likes, you could bite even a bit harder or sucking them.

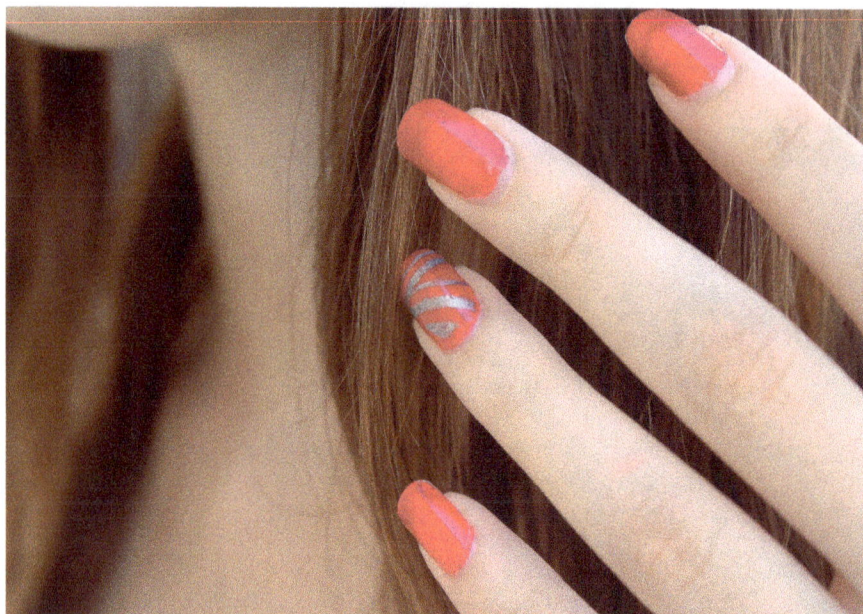

Hands

Hands, like feet, have many nerve endings that can be stimulated during foreplay. Fingertips and palms are particularly sensitive to licking and kissing. Slowly sucking a finger or kissing it can be incredibly sexy; also, as a bonus, the man's mind tends to associate sucking a finger with fellatio.

Genital region

Genitals are the most known erogenous zones and the ultimate source of sexual arousal. For men, you can focus on the head (or glans) of the penis, the frenulum (the underside skin where the shaft and the head meet), the foreskin (for uncircumcised men), the scrotum, the perineum (the skin between the penis and anus), and the prostate (reached inside the rectum).

For women, you can focus on the pubic mound, the clitoris, the G-spot (two to three inches inside, on the front vaginal wall), the A-spot (four to five inches inside, on the front vagina wall), and the cervix. Let's see in more detail the woman's genital region:

The labia are now and again alluded to as the "*lips*" of a lady's private parts. We can split a lady's private parts into external labia, covering the internal labia, the clitoris, and the vagina. These areas contain many sensitive spots, which make them exceptionally touchy to contact and can, in this manner, give the lady colossal pleasure when stimulated correctly. The labia can be animated by a man's pelvic district or the base of his penis when he is penetrating her or giving her oral sex by utilizing his mouth and tongue. Fingers or hands can also stimulate them during foreplay or when the man uses his hands to invigorate the lady's privates.

The clitoris is the way to pleasure a lady. The clitoris is now and again alluded to as the female penis since, when a lady turns out to be sexually stirred, her clitoris will load up with blood and swell, making it increment in size like the penis of a male. At the point when this occurs, you can consider it a female erection. This means the extending or erection of the clitoris makes it considerably more delicate than it ordinarily would be, which prompts sensations of sexual excitement and pleasure when it is correctly stimulated. Doing this for quite a while in the correct manner can lead to orgasm.

The vagina is another touchy spot on a lady that can give her incredible sensations of pleasure when genuinely stimulated. The vagina is a trench situated between a lady's legs, prompting the lady's uterus inside her body. The dividers of the vagina contain a few places that, when stimulated, will prompt serious orgasms for the lady. You have likely known about the *G-Spot* previously.

The G-Spot is one of the spots inside the vagina that can give a lady orgasm. This spot can be stimulated with the man's penis during penetration or with fingers.
There are certain situations for the ideal points of penis-to-vagina that produce the G-Spot incitement, and we will take a gander at these later in this book. For the time being, note

that the G-Spot will prompt an exceptionally extraordinary and amazingly pleasurable orgasm for the lady when stimulated. With the end goal for this to occur, however, the specific spot should be stimulated repeatedly as her pleasure builds right until it arrives at a peak, and she orgasms.

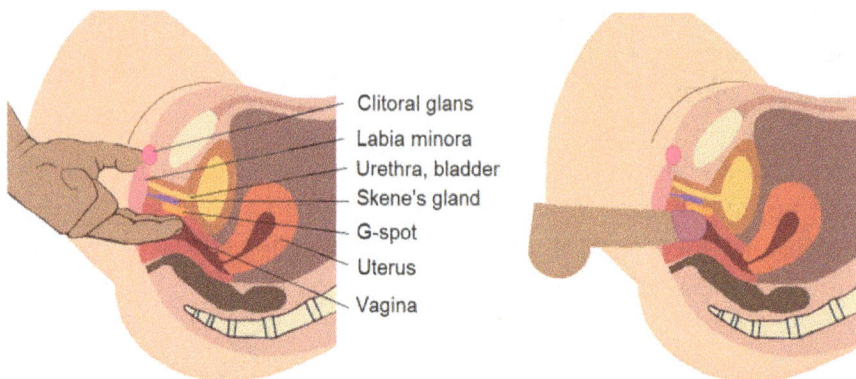

Clitoral glans
Labia minora
Urethra, bladder
Skene's gland
G-spot
Uterus
Vagina

Nipples

The nipples and the areolas (or the skin around the nipples) are incredibly sensitive hotspots on the body and are closely tied to the sensations in the genitals. Many people vary widely in the sensitivity of their nipples—some are too sensitive to enjoy sensations, while others want rougher play, such as biting or nipple clamps. Each lady is diverse in how delicate her areolas are, yet numerous ladies can turn out to be sexually stirred by having their areolas stimulated. Nipples are an excellent spot to begin the foreplay; these parts are sensible and, with the proper stimulation, can turn on a woman in a few minutes. It has been accounted for that a few ladies are even ready to arrive at orgasm through areola incitement. On the off chance that your accomplice appreciates having her areolas invigorated, she might be one of those!

Scalp

The scalp has many sensitive nerve endings, which is why scalp massages can be delightful. Gentle massaging or hair pulling can activate these nerves and send pleasurable sensations throughout the body.

3.2 THE DIFFERENT TYPES OF KISS

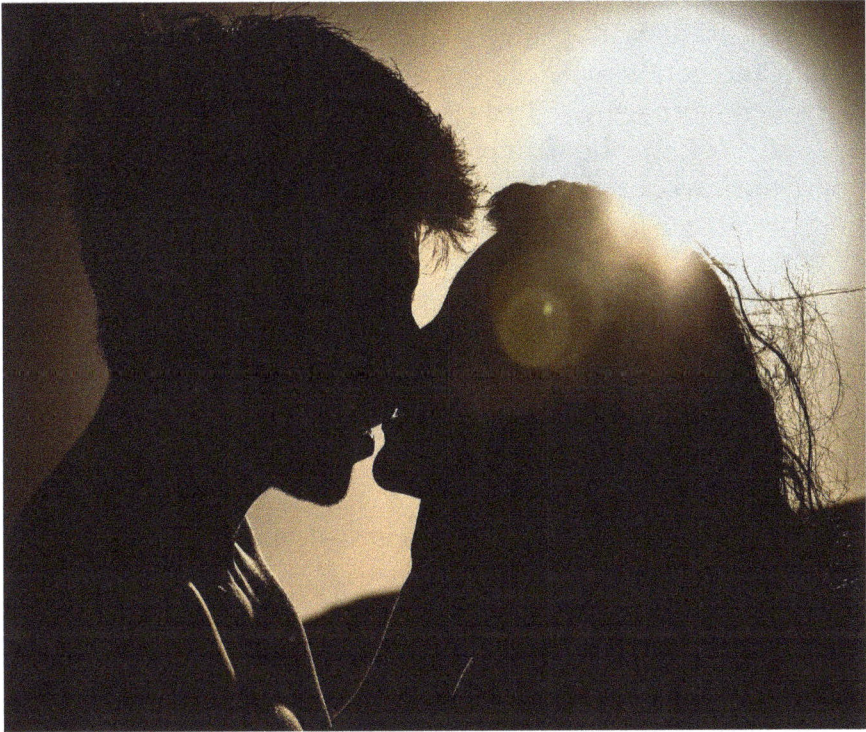

In the original version of the Kama Sutra, there are described a series of kisses that can be used in various situations. Nowadays, some of them might seem obvious, but we must consider that centuries ago, there was no sex education or media to obtain this information.

Measured kiss

The measured kiss is when one partner offers their lips but does not move them. The other person touches their lips against theirs, kissing the mouth while the other stays passive. This kiss can still be passionate, especially if you are playing around with who is dominant.

Throbbing kiss

According to the Kama Sutra, the throbbing kiss is generally initiated by the ladies, and males are the receivers.

This kiss starts with bringing the lips close to your partner's mouth and gently press the lips against her lips. While the lady can touch her partner's lips with her hands or slowly with her tongue, her lower lip slowly moves to suck on his lips. At this point, the lower lip does the real action. This is a very passionate kiss, perfect for foreplay and sexual act.

Askew kiss

Askew kiss is perhaps the most widely recognized kiss for lovers to attempt. It happens when the two accomplices tilt their heads into one another as they press their mouths together. This position ensures that the noses do not disrupt the general flows while the tongues have the freedom to move inside the partner's mouth. This type of kiss is also called 'the crosswise,' and it is perfect for enthusiastic kisses.

Bent kiss

This kiss is also known as the 'turned kiss' and is probably one of the most romantic kisses in the Kama Sutra. The bent kiss is when one partner takes the chin of their lover and tilts it up towards them to kiss the lips. You can intensify this kiss by holding your partner's face. The Bent Kiss is ideal for foreplay as you are driving your accomplice towards more prominent sexual release.

Direct kiss

This kiss is also known as the 'equal kiss' as the two partners are on an equal playing field. The couple faces each other and kisses, licks, and sucks each other's lips. The tongue can be included in these kissing games. You can also compete with your partner assigning the victory to "the person who first gets the lower lip of the other."

Pressure kiss
The pressure kiss may appear aggressive, but quite a lot of people enjoy it. This kiss incorporates biting and keeping the mouth and the lips of your accomplice closed. Therefore, it is imperative to do it only briefly to don't hurt them. To keep the passion flowing, you can also make a circle with your fingers and kiss them against your partner's lips; this will also help reduce the pressure if needed.

Top kiss
This kiss produces delicious sensations, as the top kiss includes one lover kissing the upper lip of the other. While this occurs, the other accomplice can kiss the lower lip, making them tingle all over.

Distraction kiss
This kiss is mentioned in the original Kama Sutra and makes its purpose clear with only its name. It is used to draw your partner's attention, but this kiss shouldn't only be limited to the mouth. It can include other parts of the body, including the face, ear, neck, chest, and any of the erogenous zones of both the man and the woman.

Clip kiss
The clip kiss is where one partner touches the other's tongue or lips with their tongue, causing a "battle of tongues," which can be very pleasurable for both. This is a profoundly passionate type of kiss but, according to the original book, this kiss can also show immaturity.

Stirring kiss

One of the most tender and sweet kisses is the stirring kiss. One accomplice kisses the other sweetly but firmly to kindle their passion. The original Kama Sutra doesn't contain a lot of details regarding this type of kiss. It suggests a woman doing this to her lover while they are sleeping. It is a classic demonstration of love and romance.

Contact kiss

The contact kiss is perfect for a steamy sex prelude. During this kiss, one accomplice provocatively and gently touches the other's mouth with their lips, and there's light yet extraordinary contact; it is brief but exciting.

Kiss to ignite the flame

The kiss ignites the flame when one lover returns to awake the other with a kiss at night. Here is when you perceive how sexual politics have changed throughout the centuries. The original text is vague but makes us consider the importance of consent. It says the lady might want to pretend still to be asleep to "find her lover's mood."

Eyelash kiss

Those with long eyelashes love this sort of kiss from the Kamasutra; the eyelash kiss is when you caress and touch your accomplice's lips with your eyelashes.

Finger kiss

The kiss with a finger is energizing from start to finish, as one accomplice places their finger in the other's mouth, takes it out, and brushes it across their lips. This kiss makes it an ideal introduction to oral sex.

Reflecting kiss

Some kisses in the Kama Sutra can show desire and love without kissing your partner. A reflecting kiss is when you see the reflection of your partner in a mirror or in water to show how seriously you want them. This kiss is like a transferred kiss that might involve kissing a picture or a statue and transferring the love to an inanimate object. It's very similar to when teenagers kiss the posters of their idols hanging in their bedrooms.

3.3 SCRATCHING

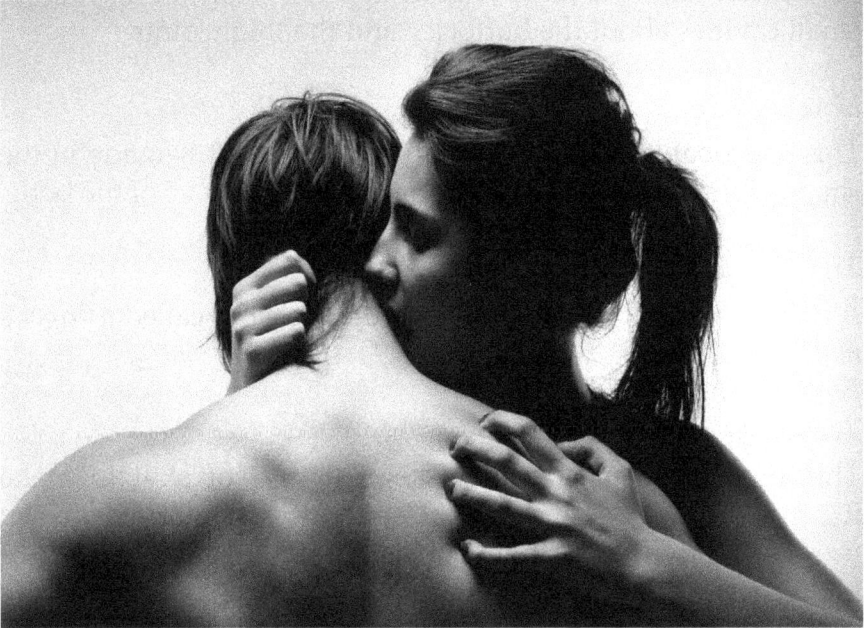

The art of scratching has its own section in the original Kama Sutra. There are tons of different ways to scratch your lover and spice up your relationship. Here I am listing my interpretation of the most common scratching techniques reported in the original text.

Sounding

Sounding is a soft scratching that does not leave any marks. When a person scratches the chin, the breasts, the lower lip, or the Jaghana (the loin; the buttocks) of another so softly, it makes the partner's hair stand up. The nails themselves make a sound, called a 'sounding or pressing with the nails.'

Half Moon

This scratch leaves a curved mark with the nails that resembles a *"half-moon."* It is usually impressed on the neck and the breasts or other sensitive body parts of your partner.

Circle

A circle is made by two half-moons created beside each other. This mark with the nails is generally made on the navel, the small cavities about the buttocks, and the thigh joints.

Line

This is probably the simplest type of scratch. It is made in the shape of a small line and can be applied to any part of the body.

Tiger's Nail

A curved scratch, usually made on the breast, is called a *"tiger's nail."*

Peacock's Foot

This type of scratch requires a great deal of skill to make it properly. The *"Peacock's Foot"* is a curved mark made by pressing all five nails into the breast. It requires a lot of practice to apply the same pressure with all five fingers and leave five perfect curved marks.

The Jump of a Hare

The *"Jump of a Hare"* is realized when five marks with the nails are made close to one another near the nipple of the breast.

Leaf of a Blue Lotus

This mark is made in the shape of a lotus near the breast. It is designed to be placed in hidden locations across the body, particularly on the breast, so they are only seen by the two lovers and by no one else. They are there to remind their lover and excite them whenever they gaze upon each mark.

3.4 Eight Bites of Love

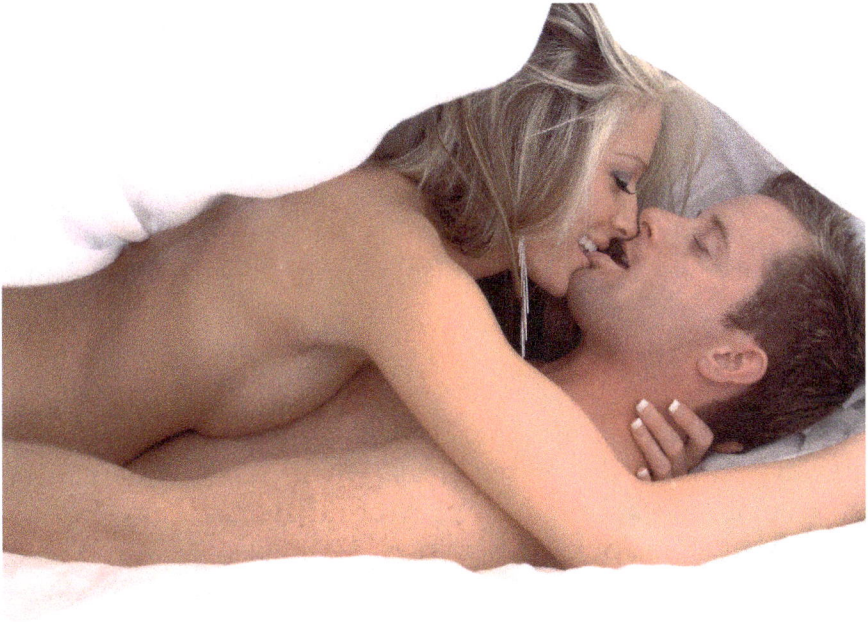

We discussed embraces, scratches, kisses, but what about biting? Biting is probably one of the most exciting art explained in the Kama Sutra; if done correctly can lead your partner to immeasurable pleasure. There is a bite suitable for every situation; the important thing is to know which one.

Gudhaka

Gudhka is the lightest of bites, and it is typically applied only to the lower lip and does not leave any imprint. It is intended to be a careful bite to be used during the foreplay.

Uchhunaka

A *Uchhunaka*, or dazzled bite, usually leaves a weak imprint. This bite focuses on a famous erogenous zone, the ears. It can also be executed on the left cheek. It is not intended as a single bite; when performing the Uchhunaka, you want to slowly and repeatedly bite the ears of your partner while reaching with your hands the sensible areas of their body. This bite shows control, and it is typically used during the foreplay when it is almost time to move to the sexual act.

Bindu

The *Bindu* (a small speck), like the *Uchhunanka*, is an elaborate bite. Other than the ears and cheeks, the *"solitary bite"* could also be made on the brow. But, again, the lover needs to nip the skin so shrewdly that the imprint is only the size of a sesame seed.

Bindu Mala

The *Bindu Mala* are multiple bites usually made in circles on various parts of the body. Areas, where *Bindu Mala* can be applied, are neck, bosoms, empty of the tights. Using a *Bindu Mala* requires a lot of experience; the final goal is to create patterns resembling necklaces, bracelets, or jewelry with these marks.

Pravalamani

Pravalamani is a type of bite applied using the upper teeth or the upper incisors. The objective is to leave a little, decorative curved imprint on your partner. A *Pravalamani* mark resembles a half-moon due to the precision required to execute this type of mark. Due to the precision required, it is suggested not to perform this bite during sexual acts. Instead, use *Pravalamani* during the foreplay or in a moment of relaxation when you are still in complete control of your body.

Mani Mala

Mani Mala is very similar to the *Bindu Mala*, but in this case, the *"necklaces"* created have more extensive *"corals"* -the bite-size is slightly bigger-. The part of the body where it is used usually is breasts and tights.

Khandabhraka

Khandabhrakas are *"clouds"* of small bites scattered across the body without a particular arrangement. It is pretty common to apply these marks under the breasts, and due to the spontaneity of these patterns, this type of bite can be easily used during sexual acts.

Varaha Charvita

Varaha Charvita, also called chewing of the wild boar, is a variation of *Khandabhrakas* where the marks are closer and redder in the center. These bites are placed randomly and made in a state of great excitement during the sexual act. Compared to the other types of bites, *Varaha Charvita* and *Khandabhrakas* require less control and precision and, for this reason, are perfect to be executed during the sexual act.

3.5 SUCKING THE MANGO FRUIT: FELLATIO TECHNIQUES

The Kama Sutra presents different fellatio techniques; in this chapter, I will summarize the most interesting. These can be used both during the foreplay but also are perfect for the sexual congress or the grand finale!

Touching

According to the original Kama Sutra text, touching, or *Nimitta*, is: *"When your lover catches your penis in her hand and, shaping her lips to an 'O', lays them lightly to its tip, moving her head in tiny circles."*

Nominal Congress

This technique is based on holding the penis in a single hand while placing your lips on it. The only -slow- movement is done with your mouth and tongue, and the focus is mainly on the gland.

Biting the Sides

With this technique, your fingers are used to cover the gland and slowly massage it while you then kiss and bite along the shaft.

Kissing

This is just a warmup technique where you hold the penis in the hand while covering it in kisses.

Rubbing

Remarkably like kissing, this occurs when you use your tongue and lick all over the penis until it is fully erected.

Sucking a Mango Fruit

Putting only half of the penis in the mouth and sucking on it

Swallowing Up

This is when the entire penis is placed in the mouth and down towards the back of the throat.

Outer Pincers

With this technique, you take the head of the penis gently between your lips, by turns pressing, kissing it tenderly, and pulling at its soft skin: this is *"Bahiha-Samdansha"* (the Outer Pincers).

Inner Pincers

This is the follow-up of the Outer Pincers technique. You allow the head to slide entirely into your mouth and press the shaft firmly between your lips, holding a moment before pulling away; it is called *"Antaha-Samdansha"* (the Inner Pincers).

3.6 Let Your Senses Evolve

During the demonstration of lovemaking, a considerable lot of us will zero in on just the feeling of touch. We are distracted, essentially, by what adoring our accomplices feels like. Yet shouldn't something be said about the other senses. What are you seeing? While the feeling of touch is so alive during our sexual experiences, what we see is likewise loaded with enchantment. Our accomplices are wonderlands of creaturely magnificence. We need to recognize the truth about that and add it to our sensual collection. As they burn through our accomplices with appreciation, our eyes are an under-used sense in the actual domain of the faculties – sexuality. You might think that men are more visual than ladies; experience has instructed me that this is not the case. Ladies have similarly a strong enthusiasm for what they see as men do. Men may locate this hard to accept, yet ladies' eyes see you for the sexy animals you are!

Our feeling of smell is overwhelmingly significant because it plays in causing us to select our partners. Even if we are not even aware of it, pheromones influence what attracts us to each other. The pheromonal aroma does not enroll with us, however, in a conscious way. What does, is the exceptional aroma of our accomplices the fragrance their skin conveys, and, in any event, when vigorously perfumed, this aroma can be distinguished. This is the reason we sniff their pillows when they are away from us. This peculiar fragrance is such a lot of a piece of those we share our love with that reminds us of them and the love we share with them. In sex, this scent can have a significant impact on desire and passion, as the action of our chemicals is increased and drive passion.

Suppose you are interested in exploring your senses further. In that case, the chapter "Sensory deprivation" of this book will contain more details and ideas on how you can enhance your senses during sex.

Chapter 4

The Third Stage of Lovemaking - Sexual Congress

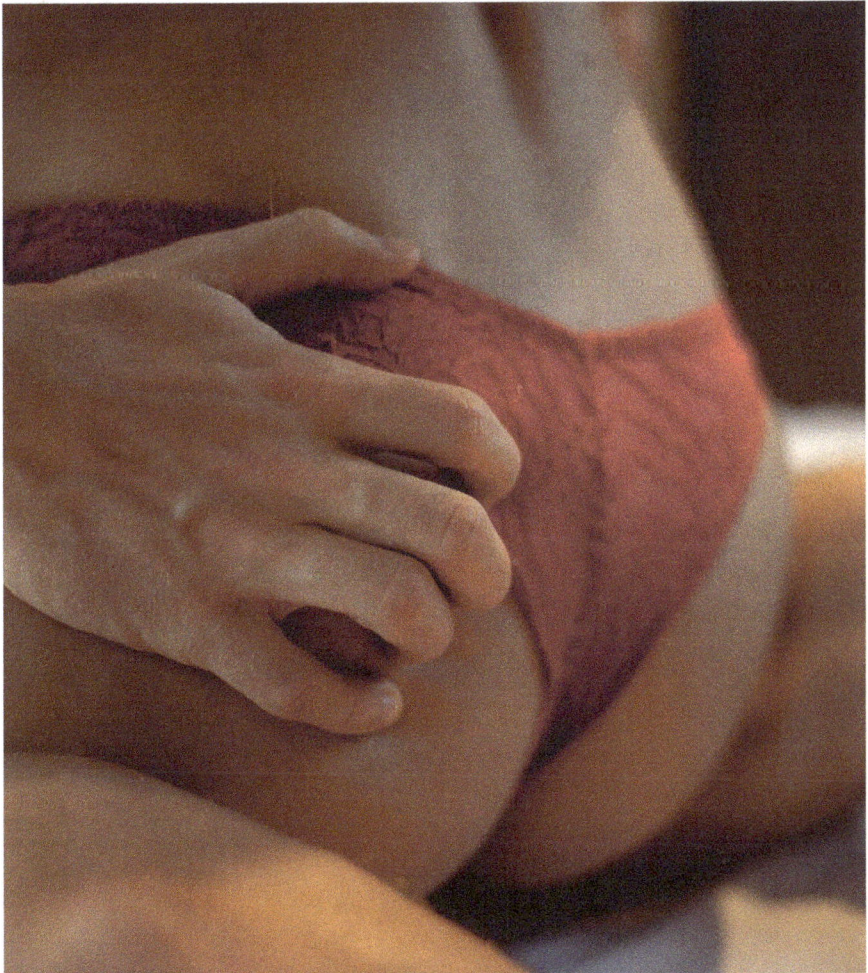

4.1 Sex Positions

It is time to get down to business. The first, and most significant thing, that should be done before you get physically involved with your partner is relaxing. Following a long, stressful day at work, you need to loosen up both your body and your brain. It would help if you left your troubles behind. Relaxing is very subjective; it can be accomplished in different ways. It is up to you discovering what works for your body and mind. This can be a hot shower, a snooze, or a run. By setting aside the effort to unwind before getting private with your accomplice, you are guaranteeing that you will not be diverted contemplating your day while you are with your partner. As previously mentioned, preparation and foreplay are equally important. Take your time, and do not rush towards sex! Once you feel both ready, then it is time to get down to business!

In this chapter, I have collected some of the most exciting sex positions of the Kama Sutra. Some of them might be pretty complex and require flexibility that not everyone has. My suggestion is to try some of these positions you find interesting and see which are the best for you.

1. SAMMUKHA

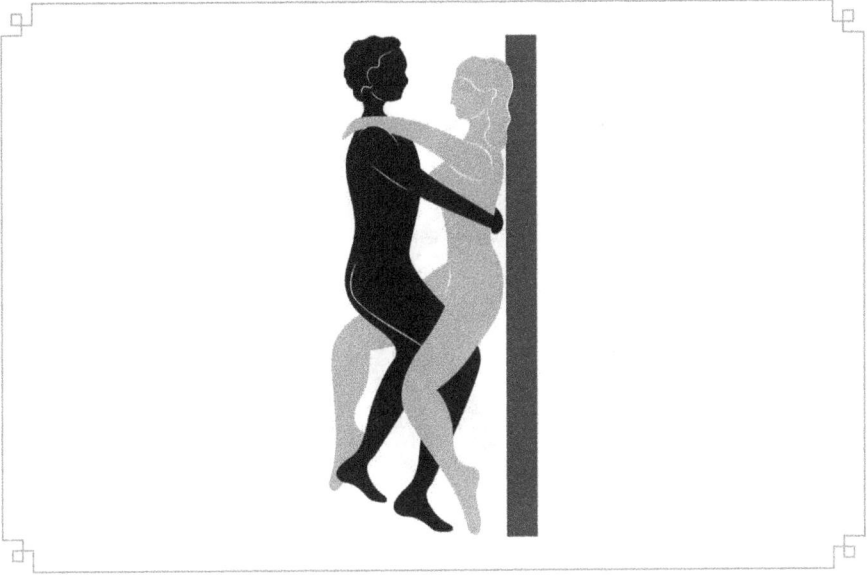

Complexity 🔥🔥🔥🔥🔥

The *Sammukha* is a moderately simple position to begin with and one you have likely never thought to attempt. Your accomplice leans back against a wall in this position while spreads their legs as wide as possible while you penetrate them. If your partner is shorter, they may need to stand on a footrest or something similar to find a comfortable position.

2. JANUKURPARA

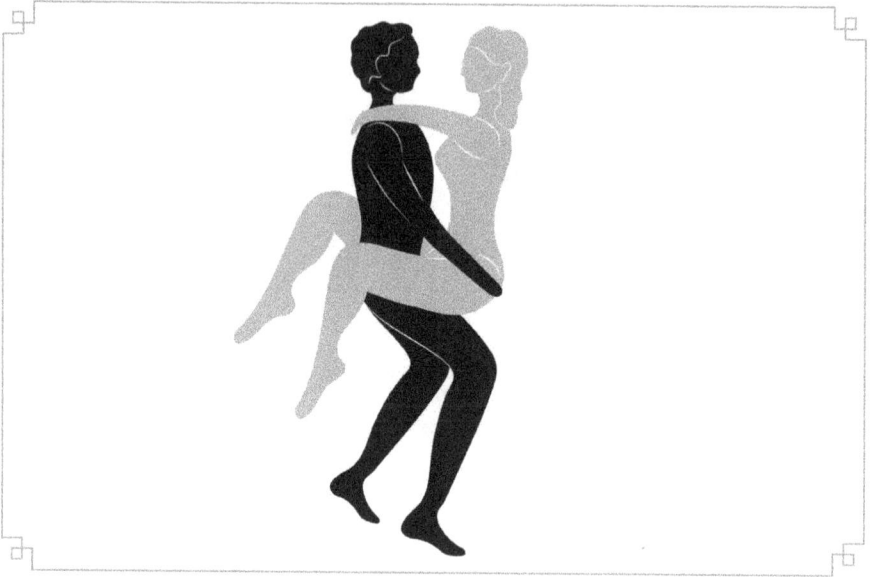

Complexity 🔥🔥🔥🔥🔥

Sex standing up gets negative criticism; however, trust me, the *Janukurpara* position is fantastic since it offers extra-deep penetration and loads of eye contact. In this position, you lift your accomplice, locking your elbows under their knees and gripping their butt with your hands while they place their arms around your neck.

3. Piditaka

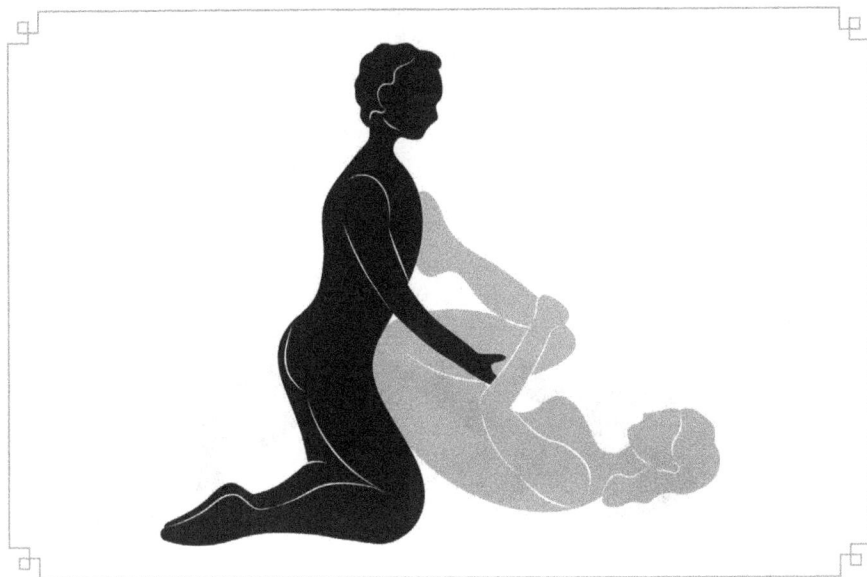

Complexity 🔥🔥🔥🔥🔥

After some glorious failures, I have learned that acrobatic sex does not always equate to pleasurable sex. *The Piditaka* position is a relaxed, laid-back position that has the advantage of being amazingly delightful. In this position, your accomplice lies on their back and pulls their knees into their chest, laying their feet on your chest as you kneel before them. With your knees on both sides of their hips, you raise their hips onto your thighs and penetrate them.

4. Virsha (Reverse cowgirl)

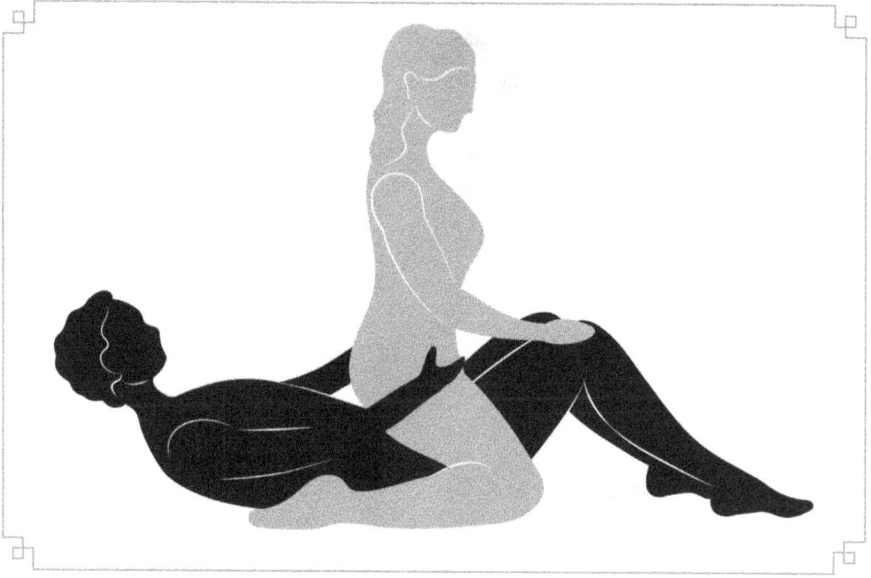

Complexity 🔥 🔥 🔥 🔥 🔥

The *Virsha* position is commonly known as "*the Reverse Cowgirl.*" In this position, the male lies on his back while his accomplice sits or kneels on top of him, facing his feet. The woman, at that point, brings down themselves onto you and leans forward, grasping the male's lower legs.

5. Tripadam (The ballet dancer)

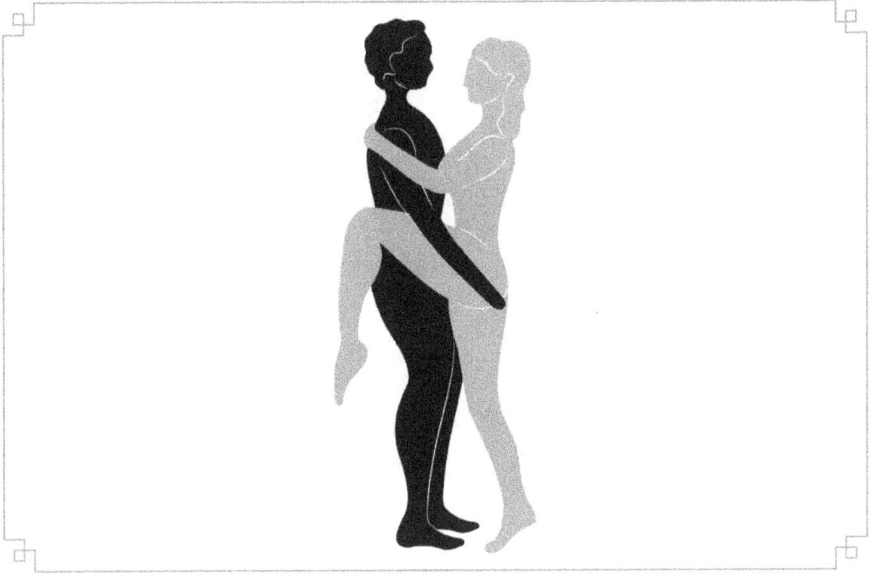

Complexity 🔥 🔥 🔥 🔥 🔥

In this position, you both stand, facing each other. The male puts his hand under one of his accomplice's knees and raises it off the floor, transforming the couple into a *"Tripadam"*(or tripod). At that point, the male is in a perfect position to start the penetration. This position is perfect for some quick sex, it does not allow for deep penetration, but it is terrific if you want to keep a high pace. *Tripadan* works best if both of you are around a similar height.

6. INDRANI

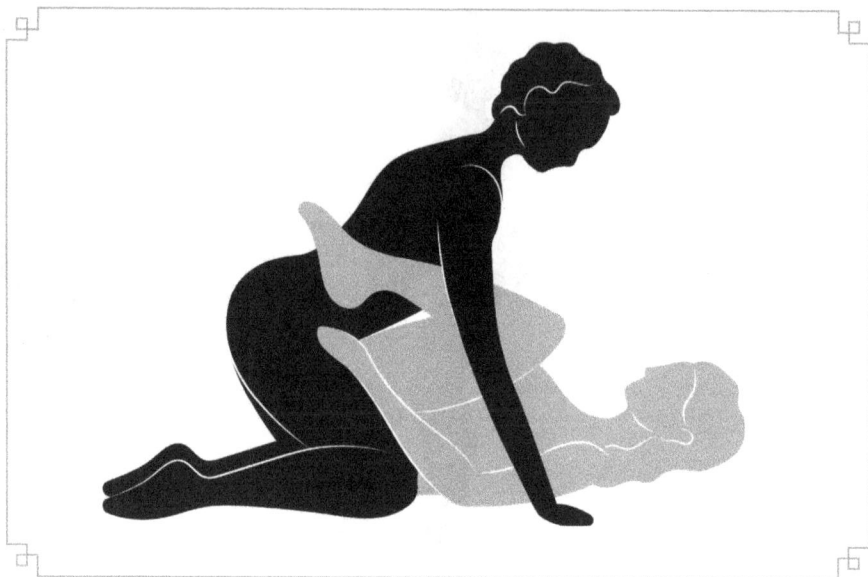

Complexity 🔥🔥 🔥 🔥 🔥

The *Indrani* is named for the beautiful and alluring spouse of Indra, the incomparable god in the Hindu faith. With this position, your accomplice lies on their back and pulls their knees into their chest. Your knees can ride your accomplice's hips, so you have your hands allowed to stimulate their body, or you can be on your lower arms.

7. Butterfly

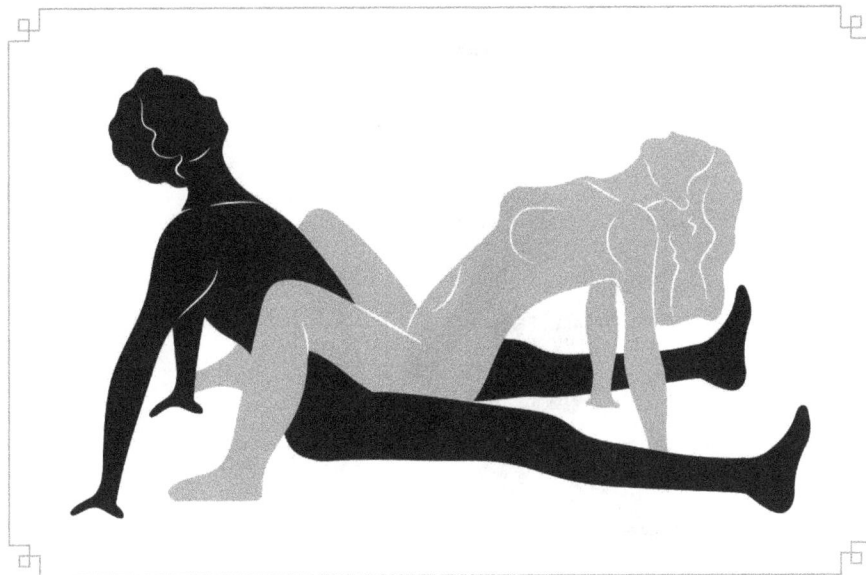

Complexity 🔥🔥🔥🔥🔥

In this position, the partners are facing each other. The man is on the bottom while the woman can give the pace. The *Butterfly* allows for deep penetration, and once the couple has found the right balance, it is possible to keep a high speed if desired or enjoy deep and slow penetrations.

8. Utphallaka

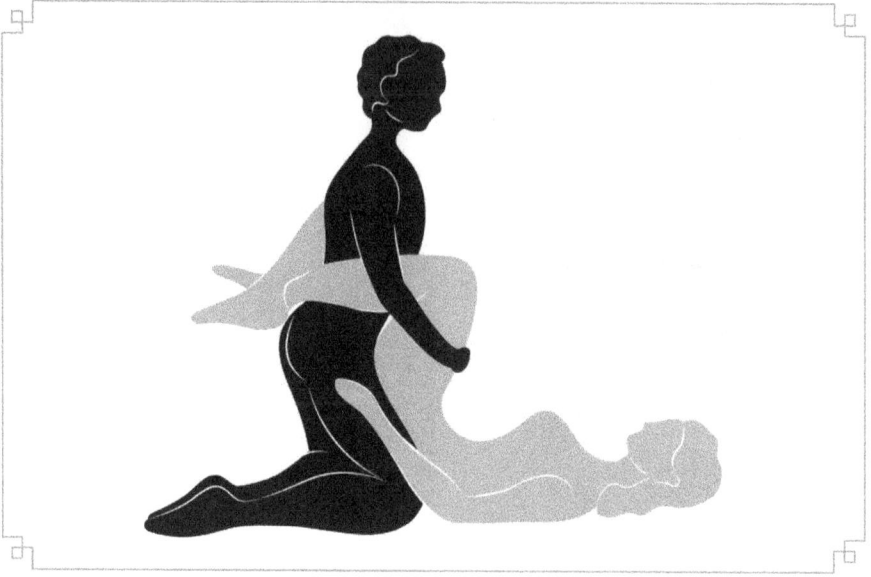

Complexity 🔥🔥🔥🔥🔥

The *Utphallaka* is also known as blossoming. In this position, the woman lies down on her back, resting her head on the bed. She raises her hips and wraps her legs around her partner. This position allows easy penetration since both partners are on the same level, and the genitals of the receiving partner are easily accessible.

9. PARSHVA SAMPUTA

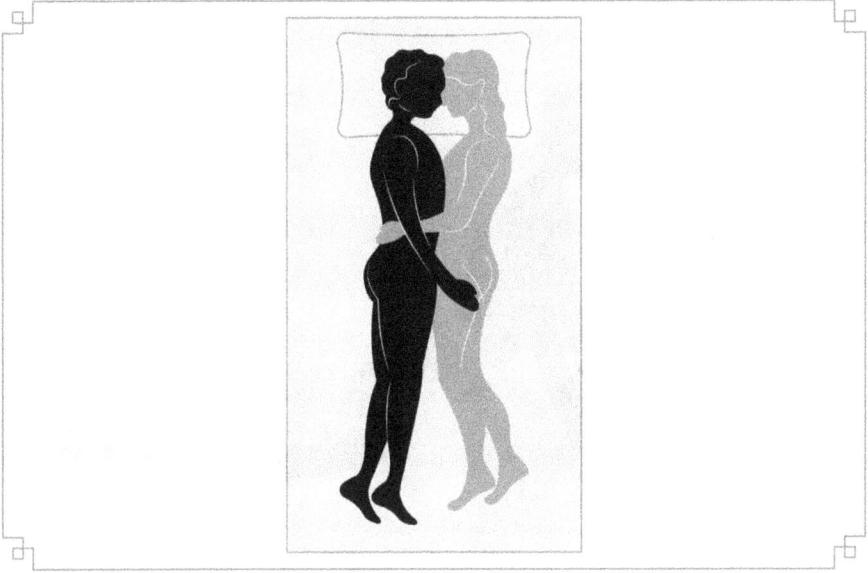

Complexity 🔥 🔥 🔥 🔥 🔥

The *Parshva Samputa* is also called a lateral box. The main challenge of this position is a *vis-à-vis* with your partner. You must lie down face to face and do not break eye contact during sex. Some people find it hard to handle the proximity that this position enforces, while others enjoy it very much. Give it a try! If you look for something that can give you a break from more challenging positions, parshva samputa is what you are looking for.

10. Uttana samputa

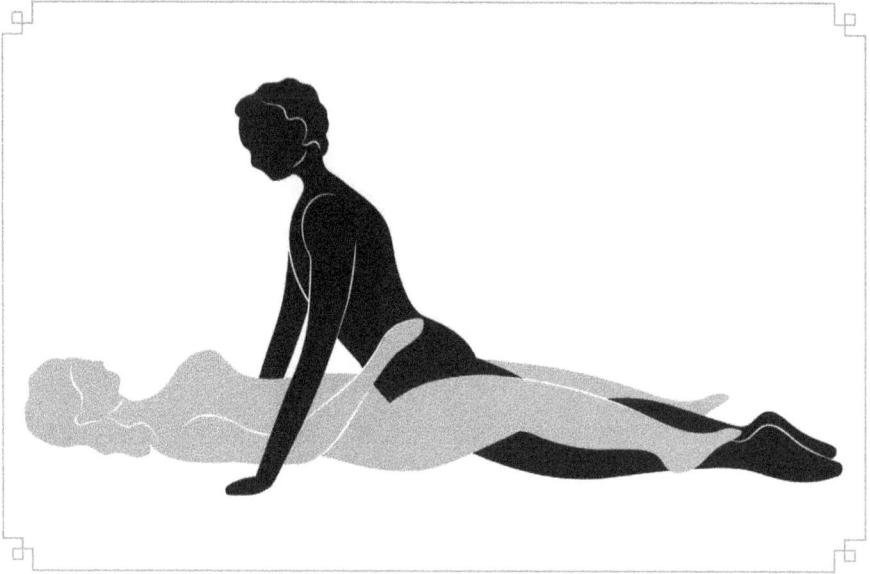

Complexity 🔥 🔥 🜄 🜄 🜄

This position is a variation of *Parshva Samputa* called also closed box. *Uttana Samputa* is also harder than its predecessor since the woman is lying down, stretched out, with the man on the top of her, pressing into her hips.

11. Padmasana (The lotus)

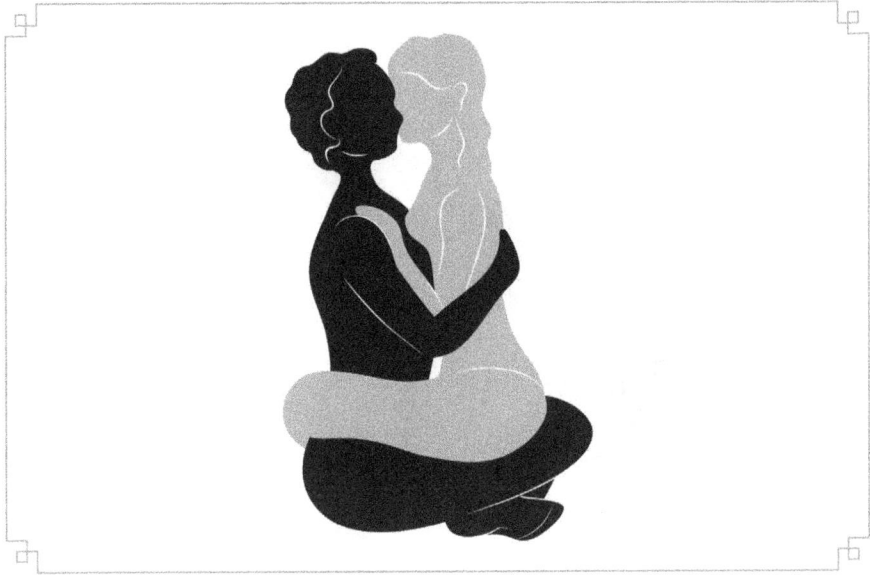

Complexity 🔥 🔥 🔥 🔥 🔥

The *Padmasana* is remarkably like the yoga lotus position. The man is seated with his legs crossed while the woman is on the top with her legs around her partner's torso. As you can imagine, *Padmasana* requires a good level of flexibility to enjoy it fully. I have personally tried this position multiple times, and it is impressive once you find the right fit between your bodies.

12. JRIMBHITAKA

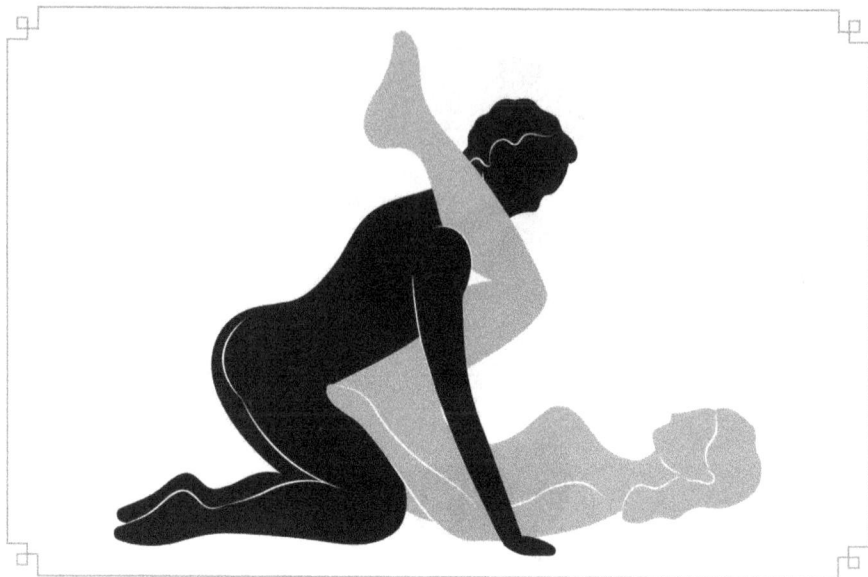

Complexity 🔥🔥 💧 💧 💧

In this position, the lady raises her legs and puts them on her accomplice's shoulders; in this way, her knees are locked over his shoulders. *Jrimbhitaka* allows deep penetration, and it's perfect when used for slow and long sex.

13. MAGIC MOUNTAIN

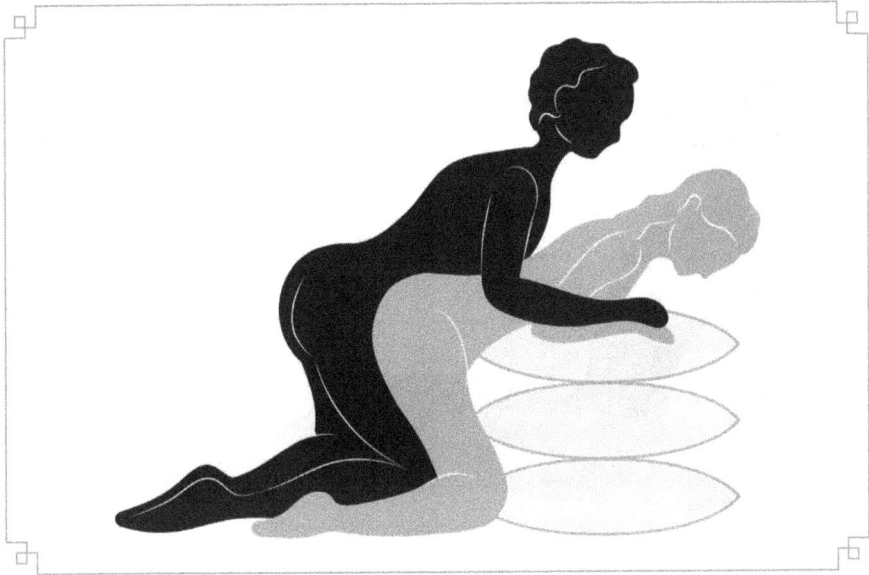

Complexity 🔥 🔥 🔥 🔥 🔥

The *Magic Mountain* position is one of the relaxing positions of the Kama Sutra. The woman lies on her front and props herself up on her elbows. The partner kneels behind her to penetrate the woman from behind. He can also use his hands to hold her waist or stimulate her body during the act.

14. Good ex

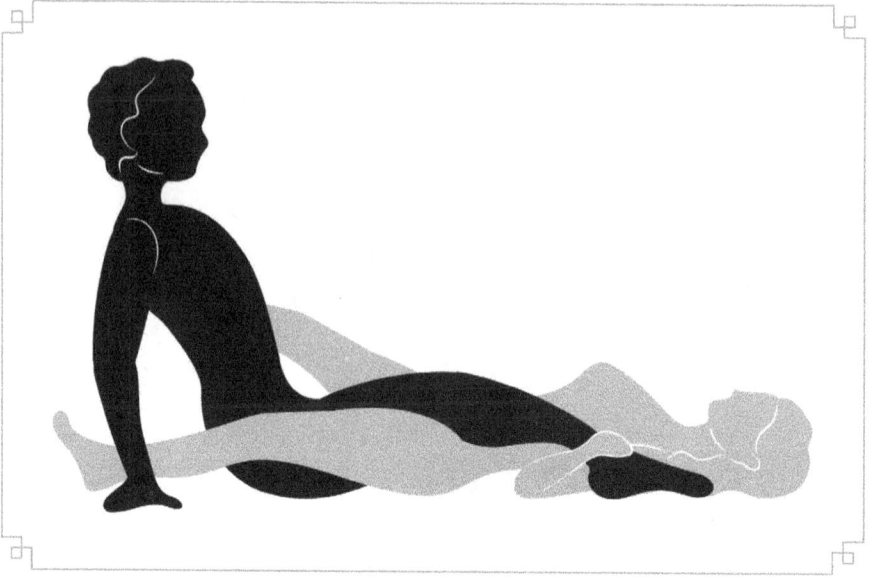

Complexity 🔥🔥🔥🔥🔥

The *Good Ex* is a medium-level difficulty position. The couple sits on the bed facing each other with legs forward. Lift your accomplice's right leg over your left and lift your right leg over your partner's left. Come closer so the male can start the penetration. Once you are locked in this position, lie back with your legs forming an X. Then male can slowly begin the penetration.

15. Pinball Wizard

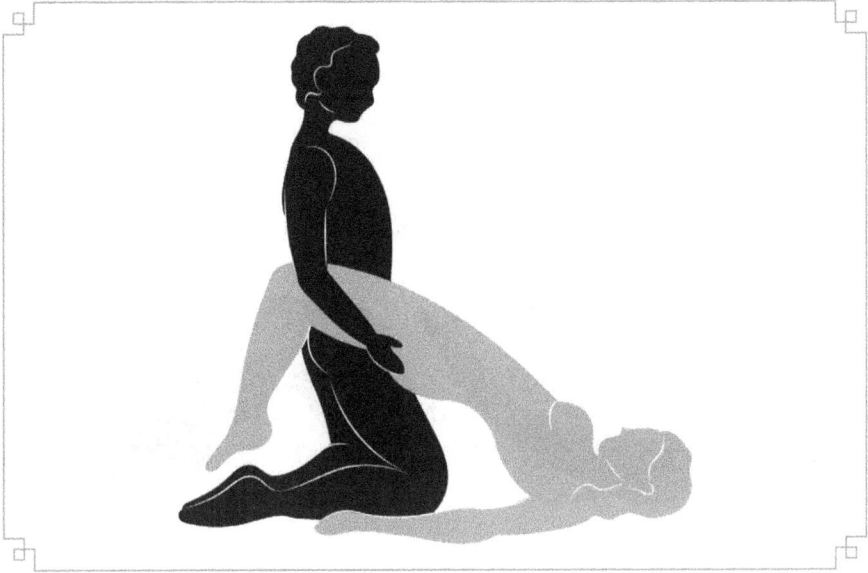

Complexity 🔥🔥🔥🔥🔥

For this position, the woman must form a bridge with all her weight resting on her shoulders. The male can then penetrate her from a kneeling position. This position is excellent for the woman since it allows the male to have easy access to the clitoris and, in general, her entire body; he can then provide additional stimulation.

16. Cowgirl's Helper

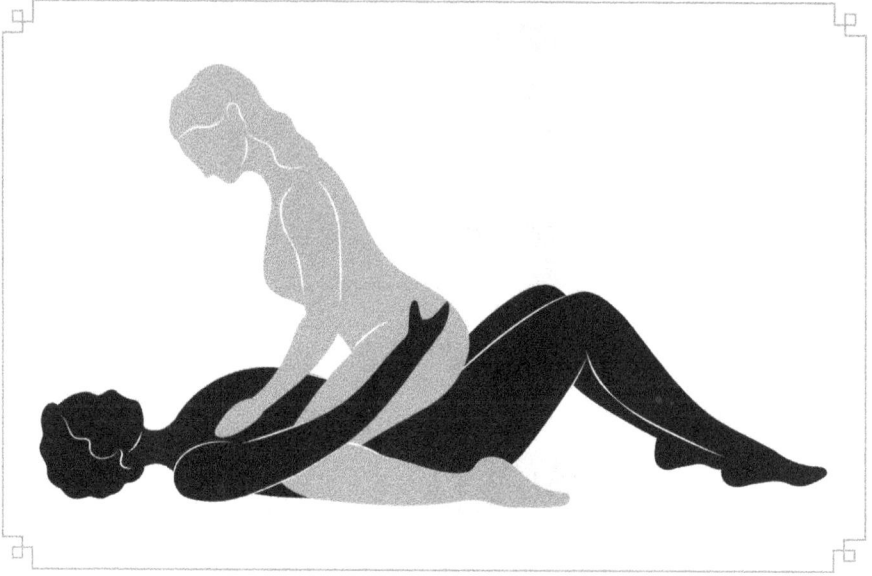

Complexity 🔥 🔥 🔥 🔥 🔥

This ideal first-time position, *Cowgirl,* is another name for sex with the man on his back and the lady on top riding him. It lets her set the pace and the angle of penetration as she pleases. At the same time, the man gets a phenomenal view and has access to almost all the partner's body. This can be used to provide additional stimulation during the sex act.

17. STAND AND DELIVER

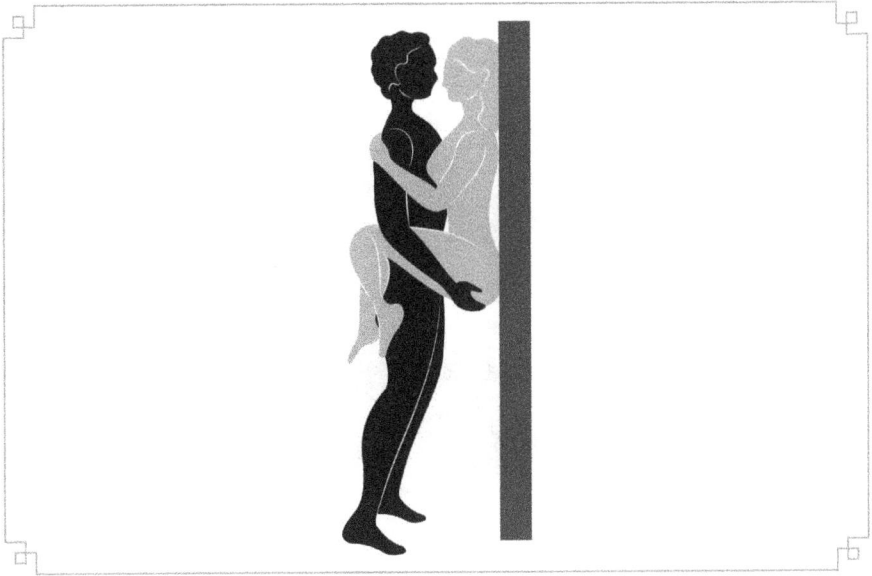

Complexity 🔥🔥🔥🔥🔥

The *Stand and Deliver* is a physically challenging position. The man must bear almost entirely the woman's weight while she leans on a wall. Once the right angle is found to improve stability, she can wrap her legs around the partner while holding her back against the hips. This is a position that is hard to maintain for an extended period but lets you spend a few minutes in heaven!

18. Pretzel Dip

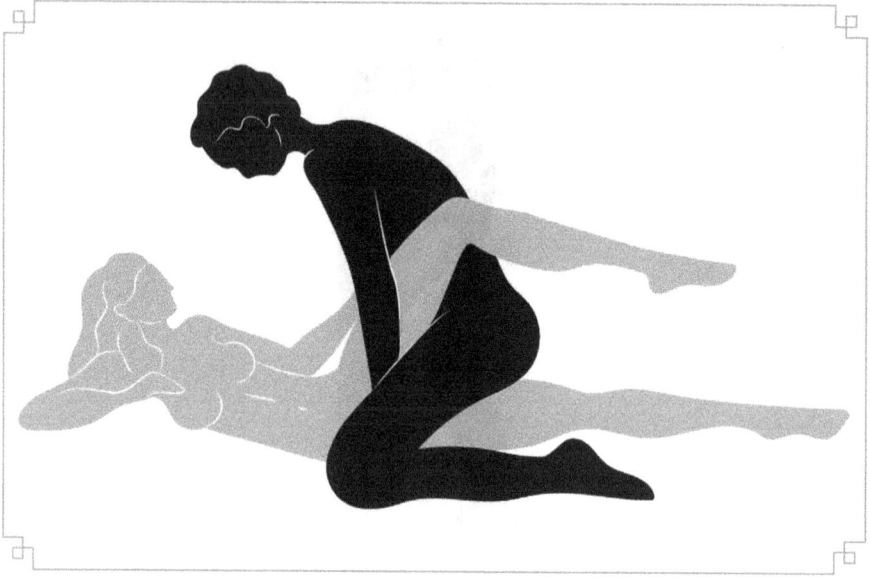

Complexity 🔥🔥 🔥 🔥 🔥

The Pretzel Dip is one of the lazy positions in Kama Sutra; the woman has to lie on her side and relax. Meanwhile, the man must kneel and straddle the partner's right leg while lifting her left to be curled around their left side. You can get good deep penetration in this position, remarkably like the doggy style but without breaking the eye contact. Also, since the man has his hands free, he can be creative and make good use of them.

19. Butter Churner

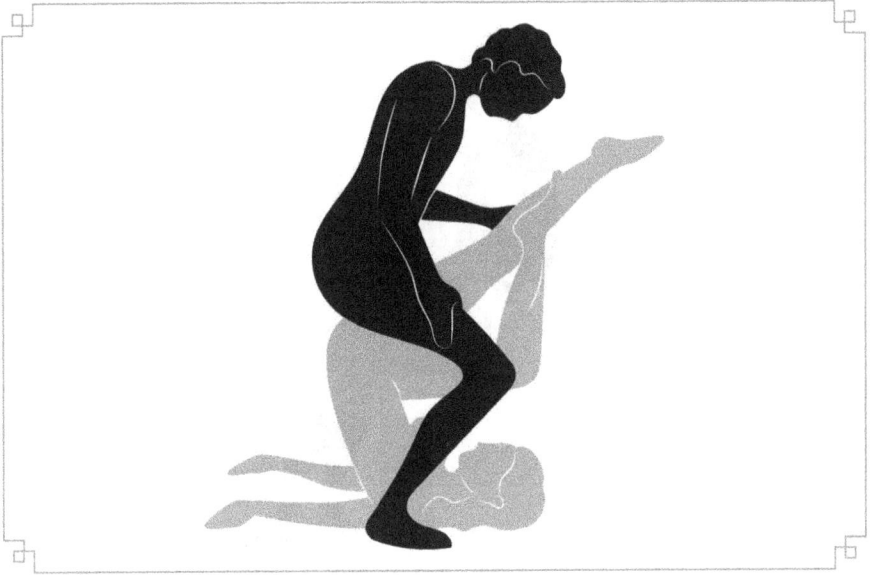

Complexity 🔥🔥🔥🔥🔥

This position requires a good level of flexibility of the woman. She has to lie on her back with her legs raised and folded over, so her ankles are on one or the other side of her head, while the male squats and starts the penetration.

20. SEATED WHEELBARROW

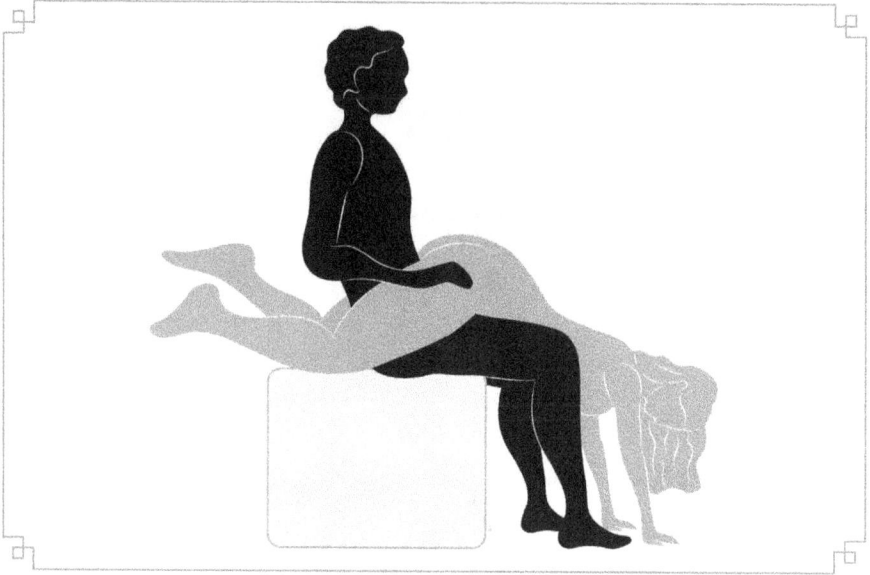

Complexity 🔥 🔥 🔥 🔥 🔥

In the *Seated Wheelbarrow*, the man sits on the bed while the woman gets down on her front as the partner starts the penetration. The man lifts the woman by the pelvis while the lady grips the partner around the waist with her legs. This position is a more accessible version of the standing wheelbarrow, but it has its challenges.

21. ARC DE TRIOMPHE

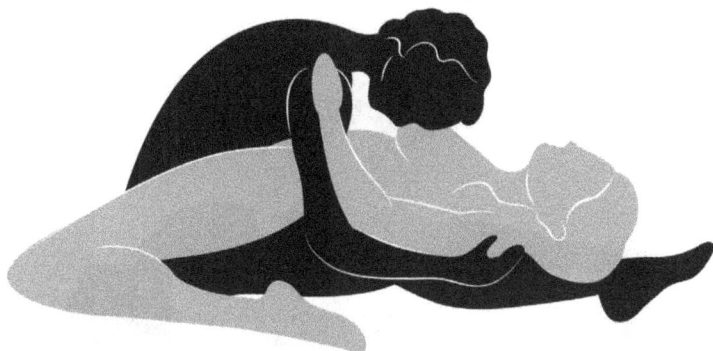

Complexity 🔥🔥🔥🔥🔥

In this position, your partner has to extend his legs while sitting on the bed. When he is in place, crawl up to him on your knees and ride his erect penis while you arch your back, as shown in the image. Don't arc too much, and try to respect the natural flexibility of your body. In this position, you can rest your head on his legs and grab his ankles for better stability.

22. SUPERNOVA

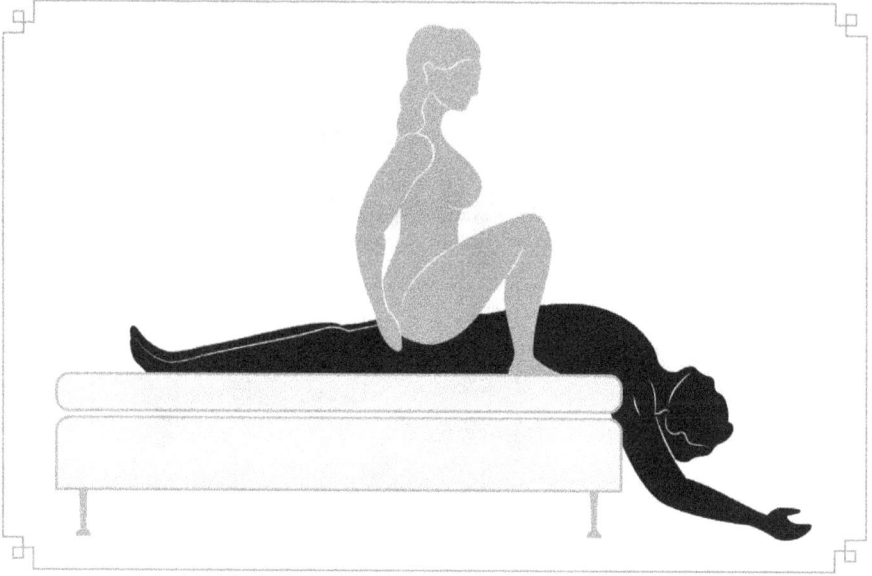

Complexity 🔥 🔥 🔥 🔥 🔥

In this position, the man leans on his back on the bed while the woman rides him, as shown in the image. The upper back of the man has to lean outside the bad arching towards the floor. In this position, the woman is in complete control, and because the man's head is upside down, he will experience a blood rush, making him experience what is called "erotic inversion." Although the orgasms that men can experience in this position are totally different, they will love it.

23. Spread Eagle

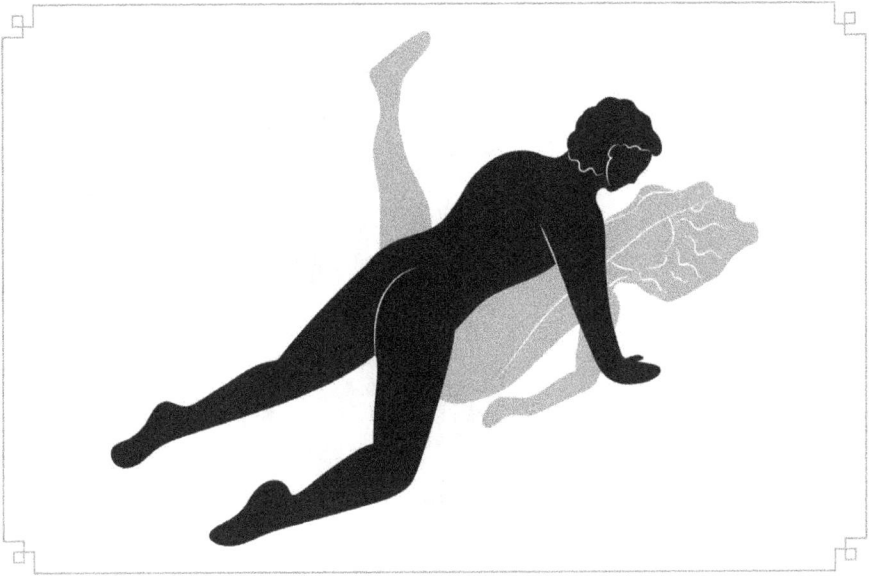

Complexity 🔥 🔥 🔥 🔥 🔥

To try this position, you might need some warm-up stretches first since it requires the woman to show some flexibility. Starting from the missionary position, the woman can raise her legs and extend them straight out (forming a "V" shape). This small change to missionary position allows for deeper penetration. If you struggle with stability, the woman could try to grab her ankles to find a better balance and lock her legs in position.

24. CHAIRMAN

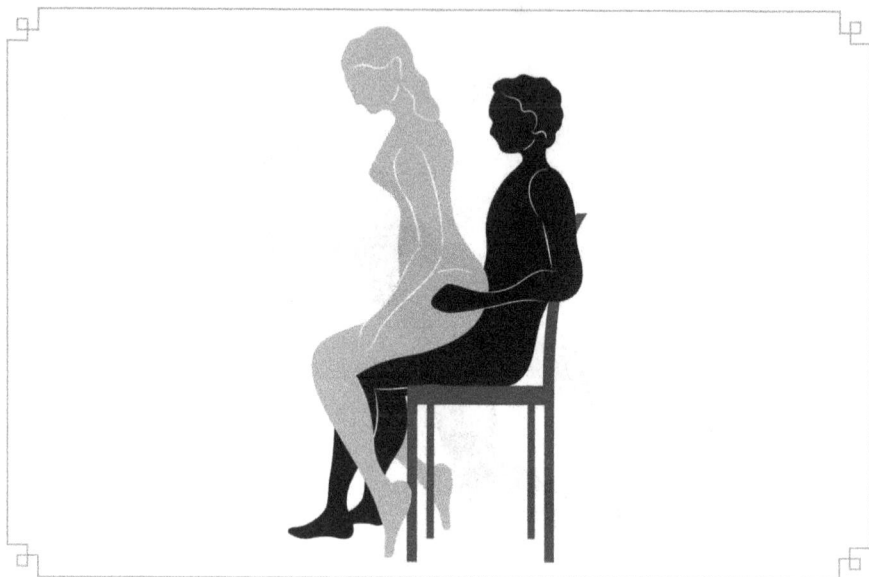

Complexity 🔥🔥 🔥 🔥 🔥

This position is fantastic to reach the G-Spot effortlessly. Also, the hands of both partners are free and can provide extra stimulation. I believe the Chairman doesn't require a long description; the man sits on a chair, and the woman rides him, controlling the pace and angle of penetration.

25. WHEELBARROW

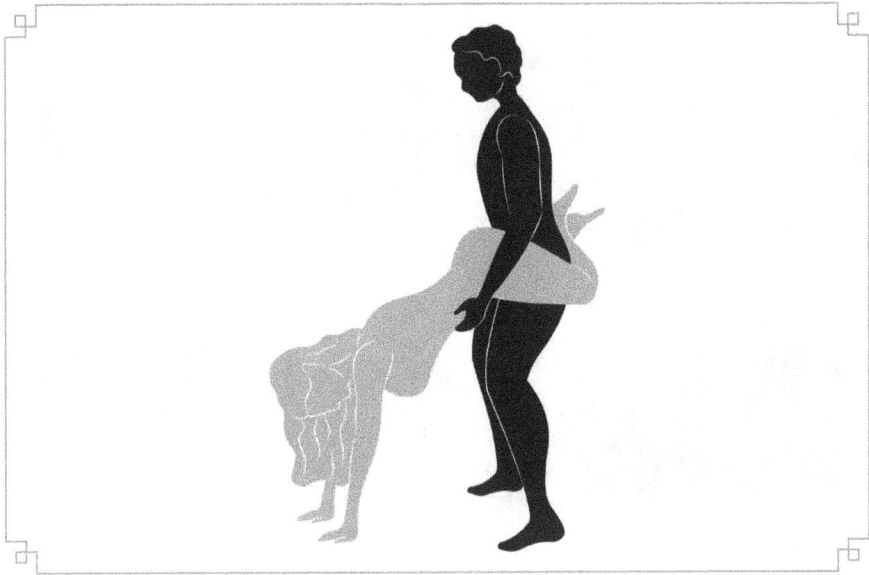

Complexity 🔥 🔥 🔥 🔥 🔥

This position requires some upper-body strength for both partners and good stability. Also, it takes a little finessing to get the right penetration angle. However, you can hit those hard-to-reach erogenous zones (G-Spot included) trying new incredible sensations with the Wheelbarrow position. The giving partner stands with the legs slightly open, and the knees bent. First, the receiving partner should bend over, placing the hands on the floor. Next, the giving partner will raise the receiving partner's legs to help lock them in position while guiding the initial penetration. Once you are in alignment, the giving partner can start the thrusting motion adjusting from time to time the angle of penetration.

4.2 Improve Missionary Sex

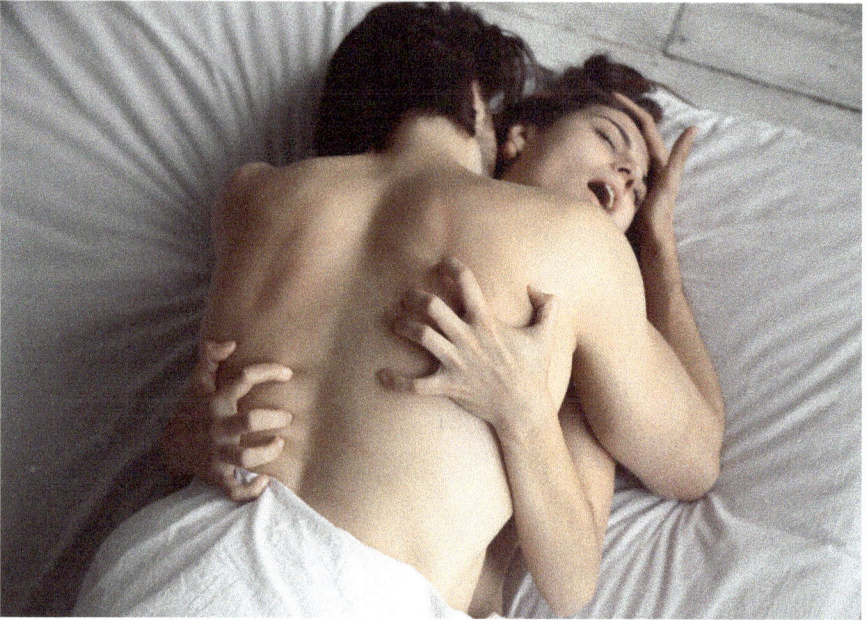

Most of the time, having sex, the man inserts the penis and starts a rhythmic movement in and out. This does not sound particularly exciting; luckily, there are many other less tedious ways to orgasm for both of you! If you do not feel like venturing into complex sexual positions in this section of the book, I will explain how to get maximum pleasure from a simple position like the missionary.

Churning

With this technique, we want to take advantage of the different sensitivities of the vaginal walls. Grab your penis at the base, and once inserted, start making circular movements inside the vagina. This will allow you to stimulate areas that you would hardly reach with an in and out motion and, in this way, discover the most sensitive points.

Rubbing

With this technique, we want to try something different. Usually, to achieve maximum vaginal stimulation, it is recommended to focus on the front vaginal wall, where the G-Spot is located. Most women love this type of stimulation, but everyone is different. With rubbing, we want to reach the backside of the vagina and unleash completely different sensations. Once you have assumed the missionary position, perform the penetration in a downward motion instead of the expected upward movement. When performing this type of stimulation, it is essential to keep the penetration short and sharp at a brisk pace. A well-executed rubbing will trigger a gamma of completely different sensations in your partner!

Piercing

This technique has the characteristic of improving clitoral stimulation and is based on slightly changing your position. The woman should put her hips slightly lower while the man aligns his shoulders with the partner's head. Thrusting in and out in this position will increase clitoral stimulation; you will both love it!

Buffeting

Try to penetrate your partner all way in and out. When you are almost out, penetrate in again with a fast hard stroke. This move has a primitive, practically animal-like feel, and many women find it incredibly arousing.

Boar's blow

With this technique, we want to stimulate the lateral vaginal walls. Some research has shown that one side of the clitoris is almost always more sensitive than the other; it is therefore not absurd to think that this could be valid for different areas. When in missionary position, penetrate your partner at a brisk pace trying to use a slightly tilted motion to the right or left.

Sporting of a Sparrow

This technique is based on the fact that the initial part of the vagina is the most sensitive for many women. Use short and quick penetrations to stimulate this area, letting your partner guide your pace and depth of the penetration.

4.3 BEYOND THE G-SPOT

This section is a more modern addition to the traditional Kama Sutra. At the time, in fact, the knowledge of human anatomy was not as advanced as today; even if the existence of various erogenous zones was already known, the most recent research has shown that the G-Spot is not the only hot area to focus on for thundering orgasms. Experts still disagree, but it looks like there are other four potential "spots," called deep vaginal erogenous zones, that may be at least as sensitive as the G-Spot.

The A-Spot

This spot is found on the front vaginal wall just before the cervix. Slowly move your finger in the area until you feel some "divots" on both sides. Then move inside an inch or two to locate the perfect spot.

To awaken the A-Spot, you need to apply some pressure or move your finger; touch is not enough to stimulate the vagina. The best way to stimulate this area is to use a move called "anchor and pull." Place the padded part of your finger on the a-spot and gently pull it towards you; you will immediately notice if you are making the right moves based on your partner's reaction.

The O-Spot

Only 8% of the women are sensitive here, and you could be one of the lucky ones! To find the O-Spot, you must locate the G-Spot first. You can refer to this diagram to locate it.

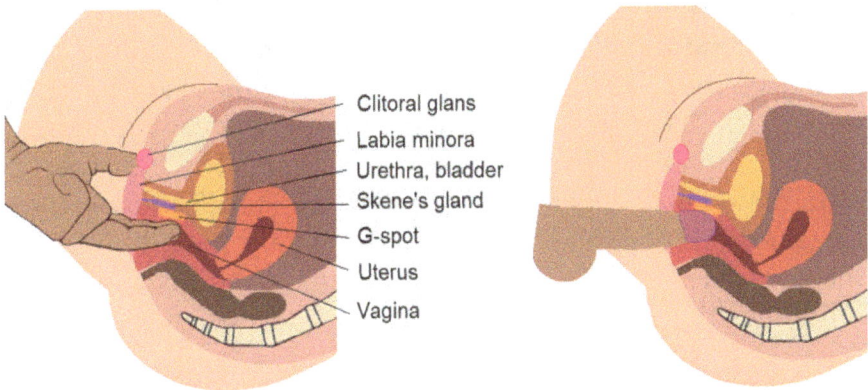

Clitoral glans
Labia minora
Urethra, bladder
Skene's gland
G-spot
Uterus
Vagina

Once the G-Spot is found, then rotate your finger on the opposite vaginal wall and go deeper until you reach a spongy area; this is the O-Spot. The sensations your partner will feel when stimulated in this area will be remarkably like what she would experience with anal sex. The best stimulation can be achieved by using the *"anchor and pull"* technique on the G-Spot and O-Spot simultaneously. To do that, you will require to use both hands together, with one palm facing up and the other facing down. This position will allow the index fingers to reach both areas at the same time.

Cervical orgasm

It is estimated that only 7.5% of women have ever experienced a cervical orgasm. When the woman becomes aroused, the cervix lifts, but it is still possible to reach it. The most effective stimulation of the cervix is obtained during ovulation, which is usually placed between day 13 and day 16 of the cycle. You can use two fingers to stimulate it, making small circles on the cervix and slowly applying some pressure. Your partner will begin to feel a pleasure that involves the whole body. If you have difficulty reaching the cervix, you can help yourself with a sufficiently long vibrator. Trust me; it will be worth it!

Pelvic muscles

A 2014 Brazilian study found that women with trained pelvic muscles tend to have more orgasms. The main reason is to be able to go the distance during intercourse without getting tired so quickly. The pelvic muscles are around the vagina and are easily accessible but challenging to activate. The best way to train these muscles is to buy a set of *Ben Wa* balls and perform Kegel exercises. These *"vaginal weights"* are great to tone up those muscles, and if kept inside the vagina, they can stimulate other sensitive areas with pleasant and unexpected results.

4.4 SEX POSITIONS TO OVERCOME ANXIETY AND INSECURITY

Anxiety and insecurity in bed are not easy to overcome; in some cases, if they start to impact your sex life negatively, resorting to a specialist could be the most appropriate choice. There is no magic formula to permanently solve these problems other than a lot of work on yourself, but some positions can help you feel more comfortable than others. This section contains some tips to mitigate the sense of anxiety and insecurity that pervades you during sexual intercourse.

Best Positions to Try on the off chance that you are Insecure
Using a seated position can instill a sense of security and make you feel less exposed and vulnerable during sexual intercourse. In this first position, the man will sit in the seat, and the woman can ride him looking him straight in the eye. This position ensures a sense of control for the person on top who can decide

the pace and depth of the penetration. This comfortable position gives a sense of safety since you will face the person you trust, and your bodies will be firmly wrapped together. The feeling of closeness and intimacy with your partner should be able to calm your insecurities and allow you to enjoy the moment.

Alternatively, you can try a more classic position in bed, **lying face to face with your partner**. This time the woman should position herself slightly higher than her partner, with one of her legs used to wrap the partner's hips. In this position, the penetration is not complex, and the hips drive all the action. Bonding with your partner and lying face to face together should instill a sense of security and foster communication.

Ideally, any sexual position that allows you to face your partner and promotes a large contact area between your bodies will naturally instill confidence.

Eye-to-eye connection is critical. In addition, the capacity to kiss and touch your accomplice is additionally significant. Along these lines, when you search for positions that will lessen your weakness, it is ideal to pick ones where you are confronting each other.

Best Sex Positions for Anxious Lovers

Having tension about sex is not unprecedented. There are numerous causes for feeling anxious about sex, some rational, some less so.

There is a wide range of sex positions that you can try that will help decrease the degree of tension you are encountering. Also, being open and speaking with your accomplice about how you are feeling is vital to get rid of this negative energy.

One of the recommended postures to combat performance anxiety is called *"associated hearts,"* which is remarkably like the cowgirl style. In this position, the man is initially lying on his back while the woman rides him. At this point, the man, using his arms, raises his torso, getting near the partner and precisely bringing the hearts getting near closer. This position guarantees eye-to-eye contact and, at the same time, a reasonable degree of intimacy helpful in relaxing and chasing away negative thoughts. If this position does not help, you could try the variant in which the woman is turned, and the man comes into contact with her back.

~ CHAPTER 5 ~

The Fourth Stage of Lovemaking - After Play

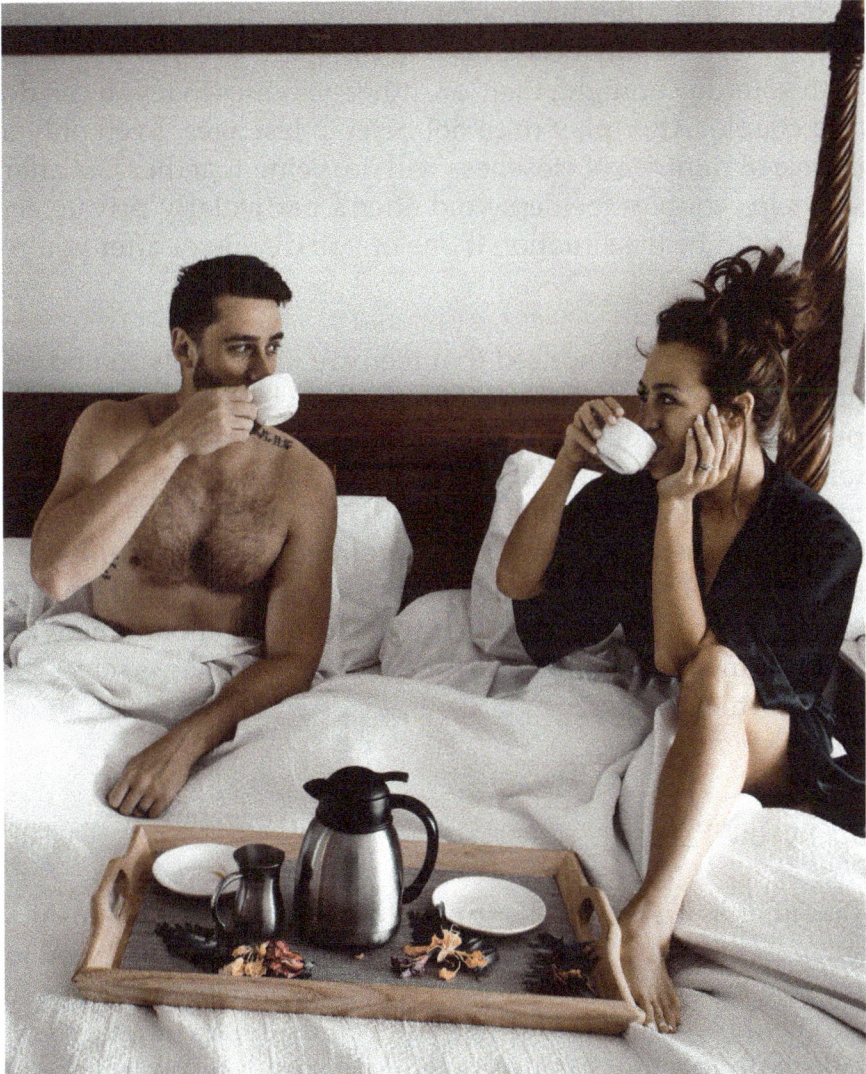

After play is the last stage of lovemaking, and it is often neglected. Many couples prefer to conclude with the sexual act and avoid potentially embarrassing moments in bed. In my opinion, the after play is as important as the other parts, and it is a special moment that can reinforce the relationship and lead to more fantastic sex.

Yet, what is after play? In a real sense, it implies what you do after you play (i.e., engage in sexual relations). While normal post-coital activities incorporate nodding off, going after your telephone, or in any event, leaving the space to continue ahead with your day or night, there are other activities that you can do as a couple. After play does not need to last ages. Even only a couple of minutes of closeness will do; being together just after sex helps couples feel less void after a particularly private act – as would be the situation if one of you dismisses after you're finished.

You have probably noticed that men are more likely to nod off not long after they have intercourse, otherwise known as no after play at all, yet you should not be angry with your accomplice for doing this since he, in a real sense, cannot resist. There are many potential biochemical and evolutionary reasons for post-sex sleepiness, but no one has pinpointed the exact causes. In this chapter, I will show some ideas for after play in the hope of inspiring the couples that would like to spend more time with their partner and at the same time avoid the "collapse effect" of their partner.

5.1 PILLOW TALK

Talk after sex is an excellent way to reinforce the relationship, share feelings and become closer as a couple. You don't need to say romantic things; this is just an ideal chance to reveal to one another how you feel. Furthermore, on the off chance that you have been together for quite a while, it's an excellent chance to talk about whatever you want, share your emotions, and remind each other that you are a team! If you are both open-minded and relaxed, you could even direct an after-death analysis (in a sexy way, obviously) of your sex meeting. You can select the pieces you loved most and what you might want to attempt sometime later or require improvements. The important thing is that you understand you can get good value from your time spend doing pillow talk.

5.2 A Romantic Shower

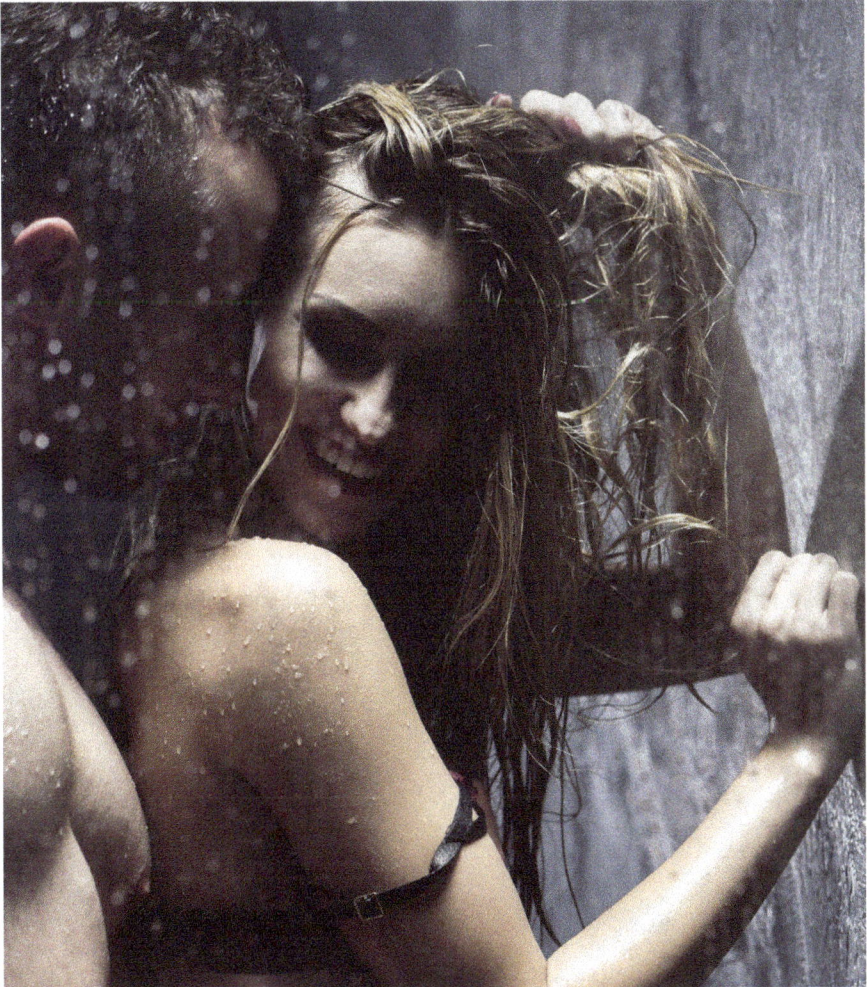

Another idea to close the evening could be to take a shower together. In the event that you both need to clean up after your sex meeting (all around done on getting so hot and hot!), why not do so together in the shower? It prolongs the intimacy you shared during sex, and if you add stimulating props like fragrant healing candles or shower salts, it could make it similarly as sexy as well.

5.3 Kiss Each Other

It might seem obvious, but kissing is another way to conclude a fantastic evening; enlarge this concept, maybe involving a few more relaxed Kama sutra kisses from the chapters before. If you still feel playful, this might be the beginning of the second round!

5.4 Enjoy a Chuckle

Offer a joke or essentially make each other snicker. Chuckling together is a fast and straightforward approach to bond with your accomplice. Also, if your after-sex shine by one way or another is not sufficient, snickering together will put a major grin all over as well. This is a way to show that your relationship can go beyond physical attraction and make your partner understand that eventually, you will be there to laugh together and enjoy the moment.

Also, a good laugh and some chat can give you time to recharge the batteries and start the second round.

5.5 CUDDLING TOGETHER

Try not to hurry to unravel after you've both arrived at the end goal. Stay folded over one another and kiss and nestle for a piece. Delicate, non-sexual kisses are best as, even though it's OK on the off chance that it prompts Round Two, that isn't the objective of after play. Indeed, even lying together clasping hands is great as maintain physical contact is.

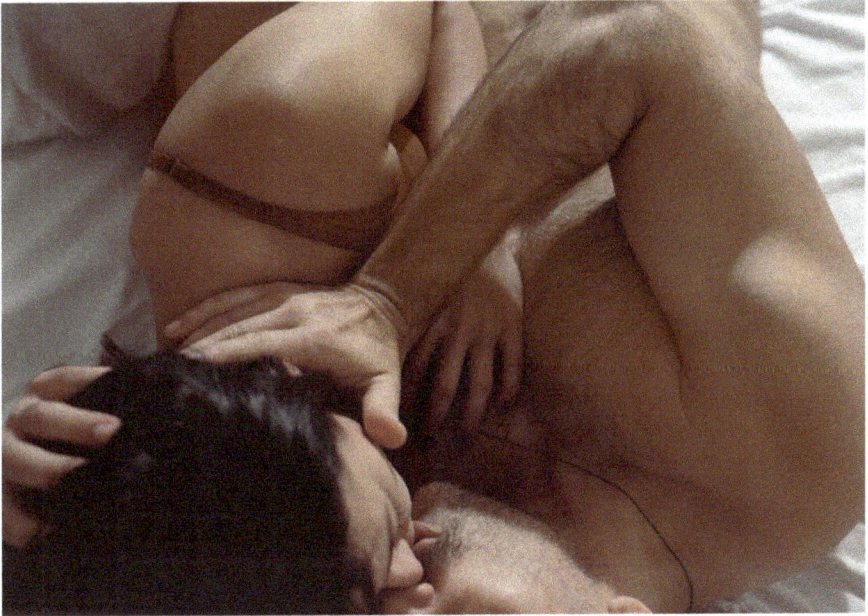

~ CHAPTER 6 ~

Ideas to Improve
Your Sex Life

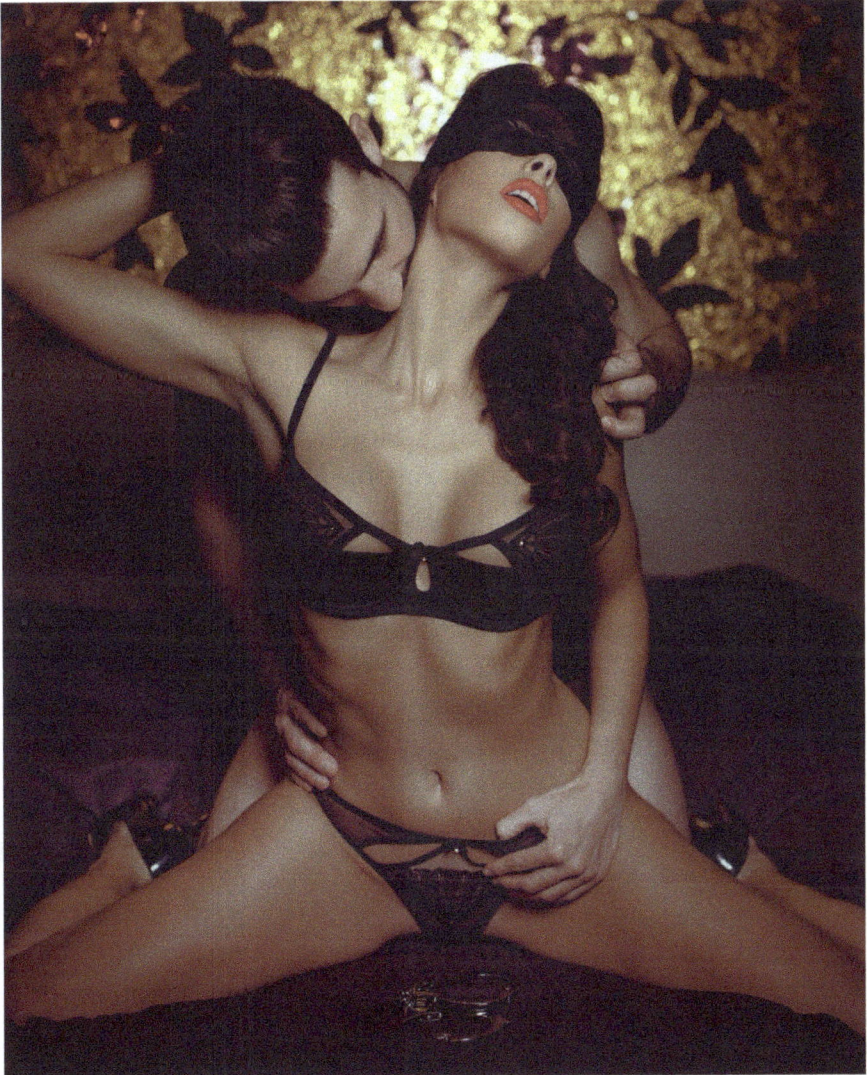

There are hundreds of different angles from which you can approach your sensuality. Here I will list some of the most common fetishes, *"perversions,"* toys, and ideas. As you will probably notice as you continue reading, most of these ideas were not included in the original Kama Sutra. What I am showing in this chapter is much more modern but still based on the same principles. You might already be familiar with all of them or not, but this may be the perfect time to make your list. Discuss with your partner what you both like and what intrigues you. The thing you need to remember is that there are no taboos in a relationship. If all the parties involved are in agreement, there are no limits to what can be experienced together. Do not be afraid to try with your partner any of these; you may discover, much to your surprise, a new side of your relationship.

Before we start, I would like to introduce the concept of fetishes. The expression "fetish" may inspire pictures of dark leather bodysuits and convoluted sexual contraptions; however, you may as of now be showcasing the absolute most normal models, for example, punishing. However, what characterizes a fetish is not what the action or object of want is to such an extent as the job it plays in somebody's day-to-day existence. *"A fetish is commonly alluded to as conduct that somebody can't get sexually stimulated without. Fetishes can likewise be a term people use to portray a sexual excitement that is combined with a commonly non-sexual article,"* says sexologist and therapist *Dense Renye*. There are tons of different fetishes that you could try; I will list some of them in the following paragraphs.

6.1 Being Vocal in the Bedroom

If you are having sex in complete silence, you are not alone. This section will take a gander at how you can be more vocal during sex without feeling awkward.

Many couples do not communicate sufficiently during

sex, making the experience both confusing and sometimes frustrating. Many people complain that their partner is dead silent, and they have no idea what is going on in their head. The first thing to remember is that dirty talking is not mandatory. That said, being communicative is much more fun and constructive. If you do not talk in bed, your partner will hardly know if you liked something or not. All people have insecurities when they have sex; having a communicative person by your side can incredibly improve sexual performance. When you feel appreciated, you give more!

It is essential to create a safe environment where you can express yourself without fear and without keeping anything inside Many people do not make a sound during intercourse for fear of saying the wrong thing and ruining the moment. I can assure you that if the person next to you supports you, you have nothing to fear.

Start alone
One of the best ways to start being more vocal in bed is to start being vocal when alone; try it during masturbation, it might sound weird, but it works. In bed, you do not need to make a speech. You can start with a few moans and slowly gain confidence. Simple phrases like "yeah, it feels good" or "I like that" can be a good starting point to get out of the shell.

Welcome weirdness
You must accept that you will not sound like a porn star overnight. At first, it will seem strange to you; getting out of your comfort zone is difficult for anyone. You will probably say embarrassing things sooner or later that will make you smile or blush. This is the best way to learn, don't give up, and keep trying; if you can take the "failures" with the proper sense of humor, I assure you that your chemistry will dramatically improve.

What you like

The most direct feedback you can give to your partner is to tell them what you like. At first, you can say what you like or when you want more of a particular thing. In this way, your feedback will always be positive and help your partner better understand your preferences.

Sound like Daft Punk

"Faster," "Slower," "Softer," "Harder." Even using a few words, you can give helpful feedback to your partner and be more involved in the action!

Be your true self

In a relationship, you should express yourself freely and say what you want in bed. You must not be ashamed of who you are and what you want. Do you want your partner to dress up like a sailor moon while making love? Would you like to lick your partner's body sprinkled with chocolate? Your partner may disagree with you, but that shouldn't stop you from expressing your deepest desires.

6.2 ROLEPLAY

You do not need to quit playing pretends when you grow up. Acting implies showcasing a sexual dream with your partner(s), either once or as a component of a continuous dream. While it tends to be a fetish or crimp inside itself, it is additionally a solid method to carry on different dreams. For example, if you have a clinical fantasy and are excited by specialists, you presumably don't need your PCP to get sexy with you since that would be dreadful and oppressive. Following, some ideas and scenarios that you could play with your partner.

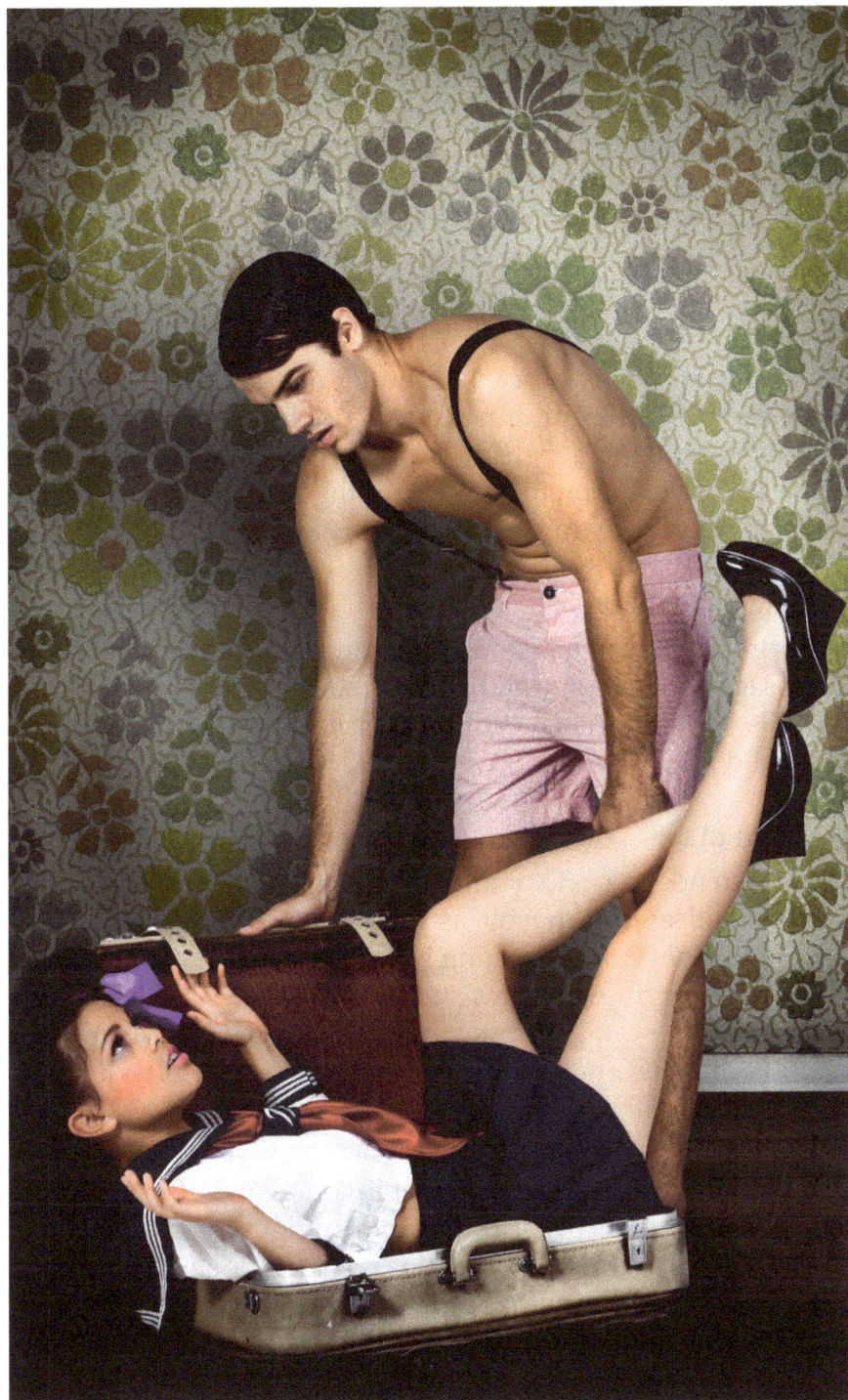

Boss and employee

This is perfect if you want to create some power dynamics. Decide who wants to be the boss (power position) and the employee (submissive role). The dressing is relatively easy, pick some clothes that are slightly sexy, and you would wear them in an office. In this scenario, you might want to have sex on a table or a desk to better channel the office vibes.

Maid or butler

Why not play the role of maid/butler and serve your partner some tea? A maid's uniform can heat up the room very quickly. If you are not a tea person well, you can always supervise house cleaning. When the maid uses the ladder, it is always the perfect opportunity to peek under her skirt.

The massage therapist

Massaging a person has something sensual about it; what about a massage with a happy ending? You will need just a few towels and oils to start playing. Also, I love to add a few candles to set the mood.

Hello stranger

Let's pretend you and your partner never met before. Your partner will approach you as a stranger. When it's the first time with a person, everything is different. The passion is more vigorous, everything is new, and there is always that bit of fear that something can go wrong. You are two people who do not know each other's names to jump into bed together. It is just sex!

Let's play the doctor

In my opinion, every scenario that involves an authority figure is super-hot, especially if this authority figure is a doctor and can touch you everywhere! For this scenario, you will only need a sexy doctor's or nurse's outfit. Give your partner a medical examination, and I am sure you will find something to double-check in the genital area.

Yoga class

Do not worry; everyone can make a yoga roleplay work. You do not require to be super flexible, but it helps. You can go pro trying exotic and sexy positions or pretend you are a novice and asks for advice from the "yoga master." As a bonus, this is also an interesting scenario if you want to try some of the most challenging sex positions of the Kama Sutra.

I'm your Queen / I'm your King

Monarchy is sexy! You will feel the power when you order your servant to reveal his "scepter." This scenario might require some costumes, but if you want to keep it simple, you can pick a comfortable armchair that will become your throne for the evening.

Professor and student

This is probably one of the most fantasized situations. Professors are one of the first authoritative figures we meet in our life, and they have their charm. You can be the naughty student who must be punished with the ruler or the horny professor who wants to seduce their student. I am personally a fan of the Japanese school's uniform for these scenarios, but you can pick your style.

Stripper and customer

It is time to dress in your sexiest clothes and move that ass. Your partner can bring some money to make it more interesting; a private dance is expensive! Do not forget some music, and if you find something that resembles a stripper pole, well...bingo!

Mistress and slave

Dominate your man with some harsh words and your whip. Leather clothes and corsets are perfect for this type of scenario, but if you do not have anything suitable in your wardrobe, a good pair of boots will help set the scene. In this scenario, you want to control and punish your partner. Agree upfront your limits and a secret word that can be used to interrupt the game at any time. Also, you might consider switching roles and become a master and slave.

6.3 TEASE AND DENIAL

If the core of your sexual activity is getting naked and have ordinary sex, you might want to try this. Tease and denial games have the purpose of increasing the sensual tension, making you feel in charge while your partner will beg for more (or vice versa).

The core idea is elementary; you want to tease your partner very close to the orgasm and deny them. You want to do this repeatedly until your partner can not take it anymore and will explode in one of the most powerful orgasms they ever experienced.

Does this sound silly? Trust me when I tell you my man had some of the most unforgettable orgasms of his life with this practice, and he always came back for more.

I will not give you a play-by-play guide on how to tease your partner but just some ideas. I think the most important thing when making love is to use your creativity. You know better than I what your partner might like or dislike.

Show him what he is missing

Carefully select your outfit; it must be sexy but not show too much. You could improvise a lap dance but do not allow him to touch! Instead, drive him crazy, slowly revealing what he is missing until he begs to have more. You can touch, but he cannot! Now and then, I prefer to use handcuffs to make sure that the "no-touch" rule is respected. This charges the situation even more with sensual tension.

The tease never stops

The fact that you are not with your partner does not mean that the *"tease and denial"* stops. A phone is enough to drive your partner crazy and make sure that sexual tension builds throughout the day. Send your partner some nudes while you are both at work, leave a sexy voice message or try some phone sex during lunch break. If the fear of being caught red-handed excites you, why not try to assign some tasks to your partner to be carried out in a public place? I like to send my man some nudes and ask him to find a private place at work to masturbate. Of course, he can not cum, but he must go as close to orgasm as possible. This is called edging, and trust me, when he gets home in the evening, he only has one thing on his mind.

Do you really need panties?

Try to do housework without panties or if you feel more adventurous, go for a walk in a public place and forget your panties at home. Then, flash him "accidentally" when he least expects it. You could also go further and ask your partner to give you oral pleasure but without reciprocating.
I remember one year when we went camping, my man's tongue has never been so busy in his entire life.

Masturbate in front of your partner

A much more straightforward way to turn your partner on is to masturbate in front of him. He will be faced with what he craves most, but you can deny him from reaching it.

Start a quick makeout or oral sex session

If you want to go further, then start a quickie; the important thing is to stop before the point of no return. The same criteria can be applied to oral sex. You can slowly excite your partner, just enough to get his engine running, and then stop before he takes off.

6.3 Bondage

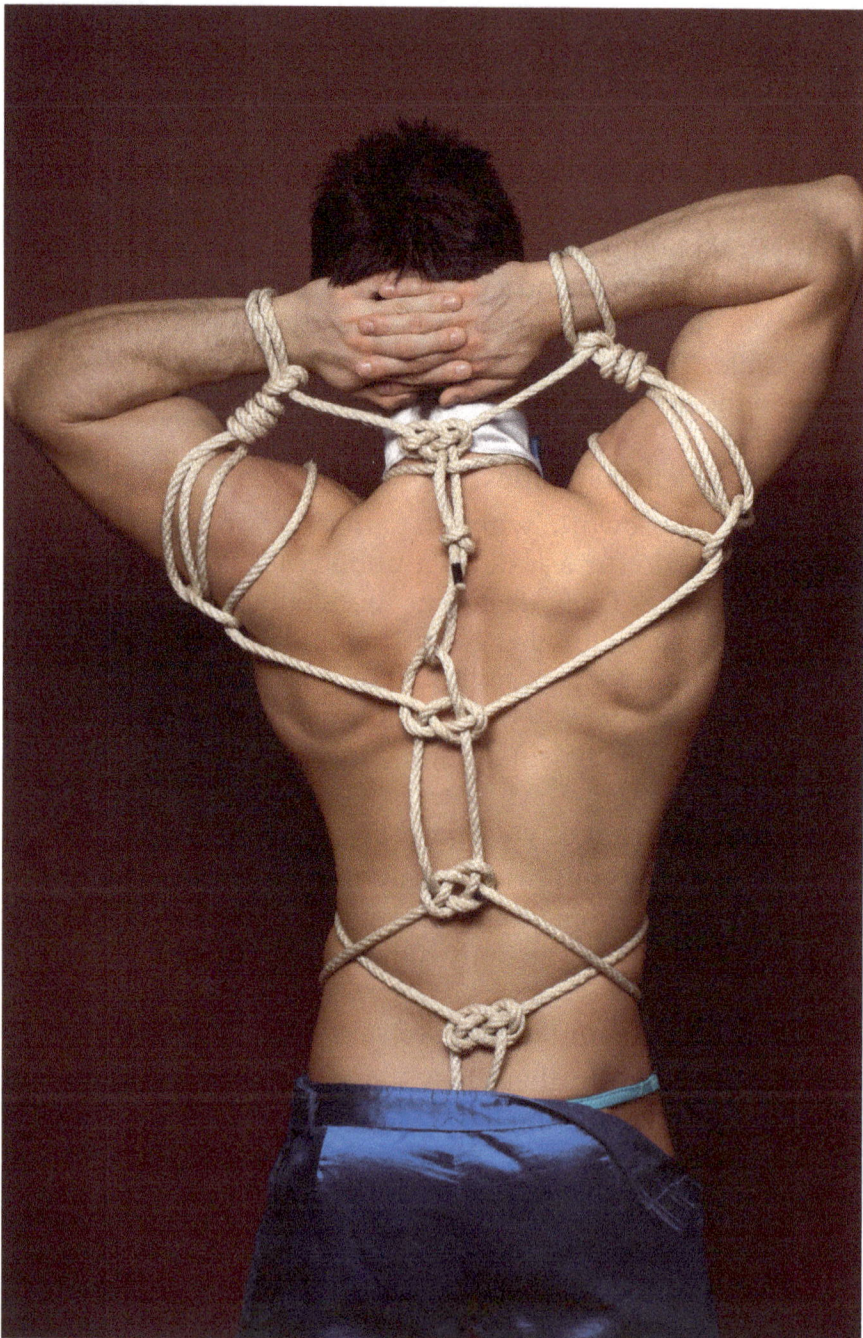

Bondage is a common fantasy, and it represents the B in BDSM (Bondage, Discipline, Sadism, and Masochism).

Wikipedia has a great definition of bondage:

"...is the practice of consensually tying, binding, or restraining a partner for erotic, aesthetic, or somatosensory stimulation. It means the need to tie someone up or be tied up. A partner may be physically restrained in a variety of ways, including the use of rope, cuffs, bondage tape, or self-adhering bandage."

So many people incorporate different levels of bondage into their sex lives; think about how many models of fluffy handcuffs there are around. Going deep into the topic would require a book of its own. What I would try to do in this section is giving you some basic principles and ideas that you can try with your partner.

If both of you are interested in this practice, I would suggest you buy a book dedicated solely to the subject and/or watch the various video tutorials available online. Whether you are an expert or a novice, it is essential to approach this technique as safely as possible. These are basic safety guidelines that you should always follow:

- **Use a safeword** or some clear way for the bound partner to stop the game.
- **Never leaving a bound person alone**.
- To avoid circulation problems, make sure that the bound person changes positions at least once an hour.
- Make sure that you can quickly release the bound person in case of an emergency.
- **Avoid restraints that impair breathing**.
- **Have scissors on hand** in case of a problem that requires cutting a rope.

Following, a few beginners' ideas you could try.

1. Beginner's Luck

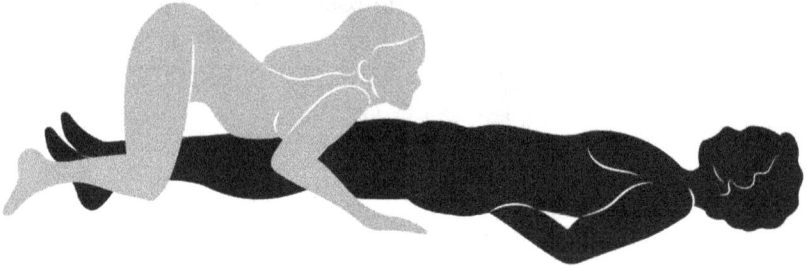

With this, you can avoid using ropes and feel bound. It is perfect if you want to give it a try but not fully commit. One of the partners lies on the bed with the hands behind their back. The other person can have fun, having their disposal of the fully exposed partner's body.

2. THE FULL SPREAD

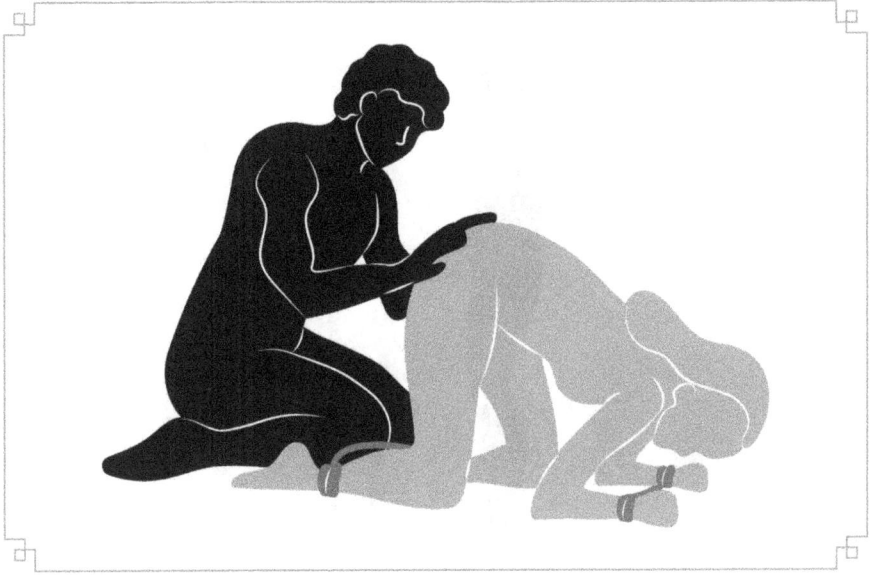

You will need a spreader bar or just some bondage tape and a broom handle for this position.

The receiver is in all fours with the bar attached to the ankles. This forces the receiver's ankles apart and gives easy access to their butt. In this position, the giver can be creative and use toys, mouth, hands, or penetration to stimulate the receiver.

3. The Naughty Chair

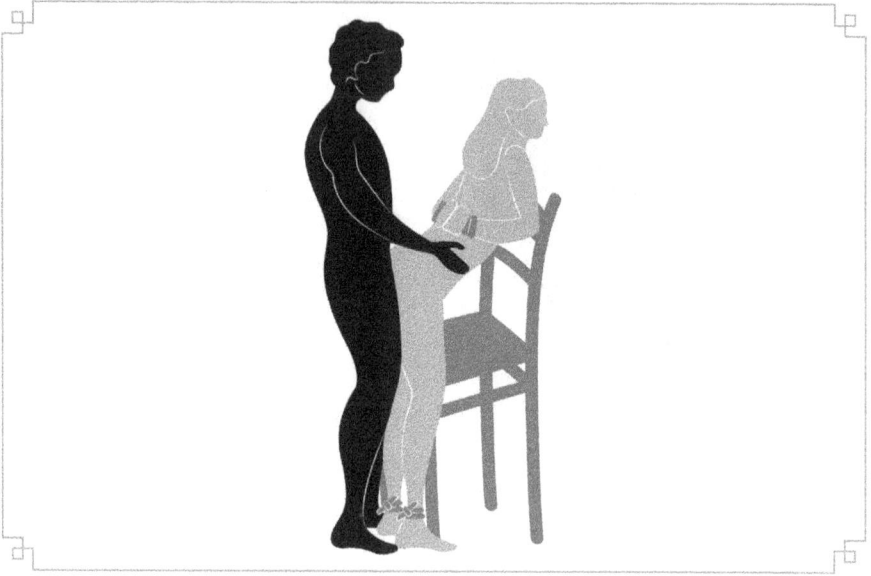

For this position, you will require three pieces of rope that will be used to secure the receiver to *"The Naughty Chair."* First, the receiver sits backward on a hard, armless chair. The receiver then stands leaning on the back of the chair while their butt hangs over the front edge. Next, the first two pieces of ropes are used to bind the receiver ankles to the front chair legs. To complete the opera, the receiver's hands are tied behind the back with the third. This position is perfect for some roleplay situations and anal sex. It also allows for a quick release and causes only slight discomfort.

4. The X Factor

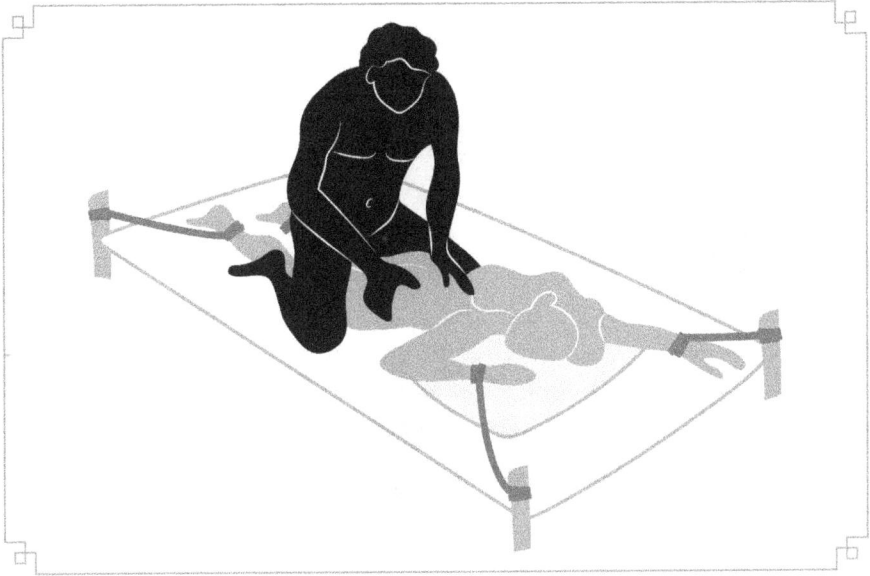

This position requires four pieces of rope or, if you want to go pro, you can buy are under the bed restraint system. The receiver lies on the bed in a face-down position. Arms and legs are tied to the corners of the bed so that the receiver's body forms an X. This position is perfect for beginners since it is incredibly comfortable and being face down feels less exposing.

5. PASS THE VELVET ROPE

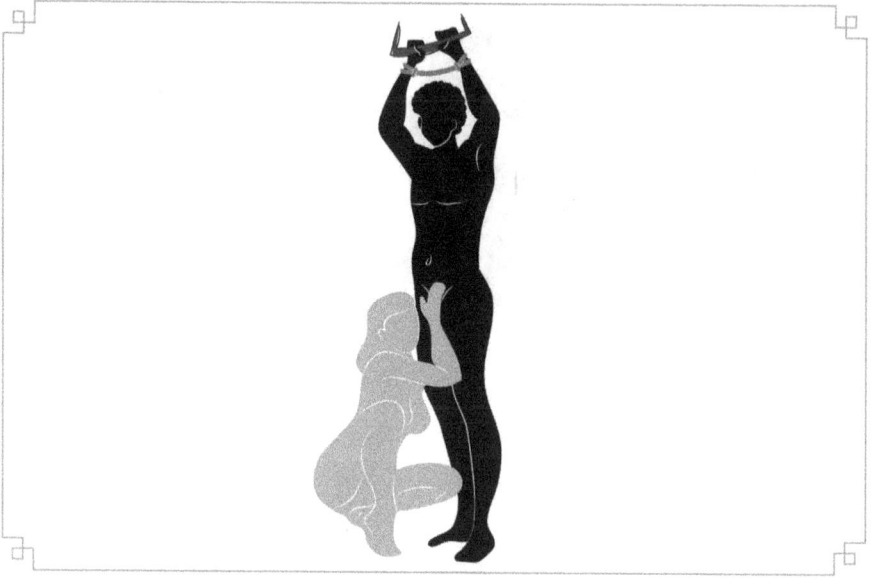

This position can be achieved both in a standing and lying position. For a standing position, you can use restraints that fit over a door. Depending on your preferences, you could position the receiver's back against the door or towards you. If you decide to adopt the standing position, then the receiver's wrists are secured over the head to the door. If you choose to use the lying position, then the wrists are tied to the bed's headboard. In both cases, the genitals or butt, depending on which direction the receiver is facing, are exposed. You could try to use only your mouth to touch the receiver's body, or you might have different ideas!

6. ON THE ROPES

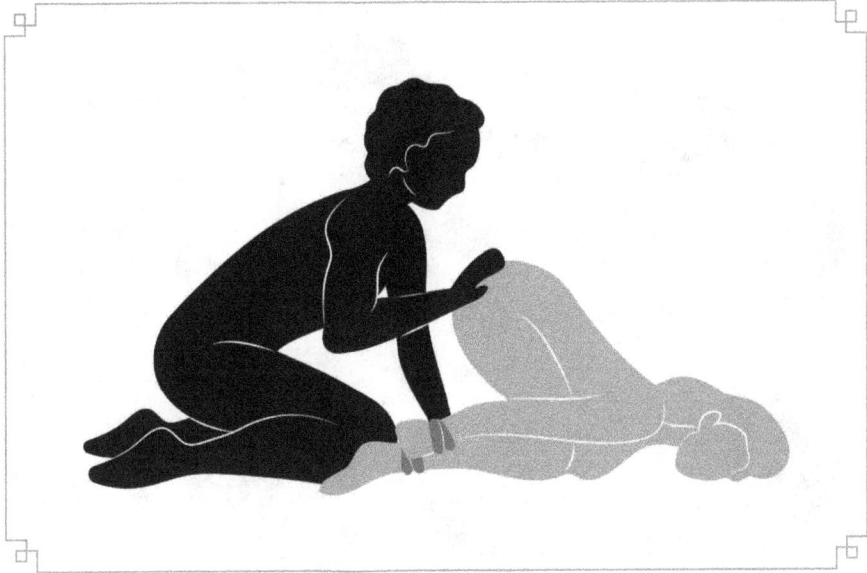

In this position, the receiver kneels with their face on the bed. The left Ankle is tied to the left wrist, and the right ankle is linked to the right wrist in a position that resembles doggy style. This position is perfect for anal play since the receiver's bum is completely exposed, but it can be used, also, for amazing handjobs. In a variation of this position, the receiver is lying on the back and is bound precisely in the same way. In this way, the genitals of the receiver are entirely exposed to the giver's attention.

6.4 Foot Fetish

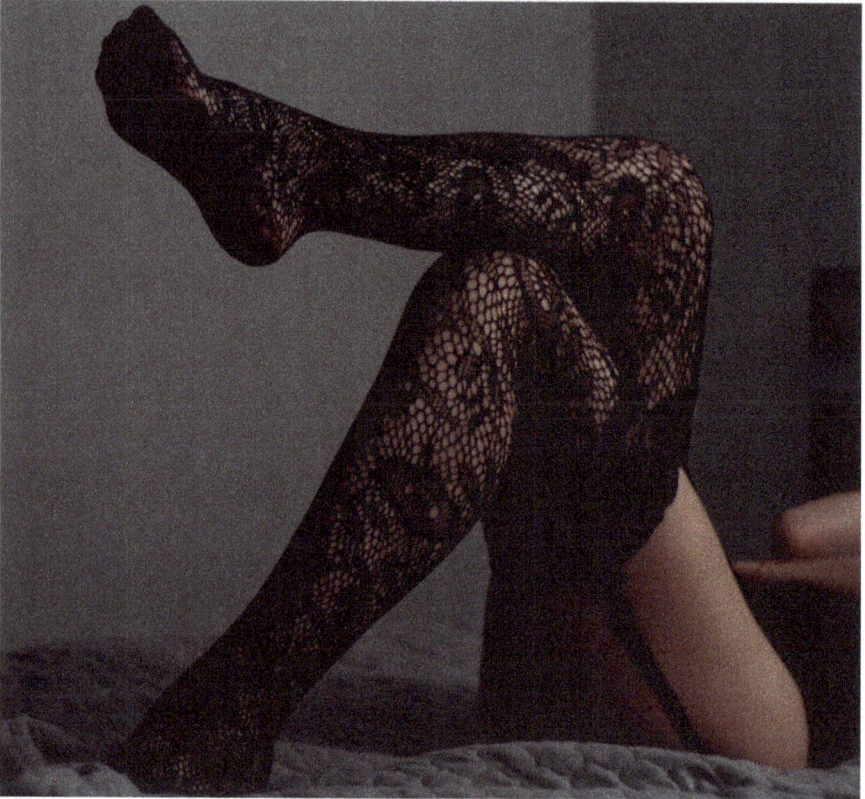

Academic studies have found that feet and foot accessories are the most fetishized of all non-genital body parts and objects. Nearly half of all such fetishes focus on feet, and almost two-thirds of fetishes for objects associated with the body are for shoes and socks. The most probable reason for that has been found in the fact that the areas of the brain related to genitals and feet are adjacent. Therefore, a lot of people have their brains wired in a way that they find feet sexy! If you or your partner are among them, it is worth discussing the topic and exploring the idea. Of course, there is nothing wrong with being attracted from parts of the body other than the genitals, buttocks, or breasts. However, taboos are finally starting to break down in today's society, and a person should not be ashamed to discuss his sexual urges with the person he loves. Feet are sexy and can be incorporated into your games. Try to wear a nice pair of heels and nice stockings, and use your extremities to massage your partner's body, including the genitals.

Besides, kissing the feet and licking the toes is a common practice that can be included in the foreplay.

6.5 Spanking

Spanking is an ancient practice; earlier depictions of erotic spanking can be found in the Etruscan Tomb of the Whipping from the fifth century BC. This practice was present in the original Kama Sutra (400 BC), which suggested its use to enhance sexual arousal. The 20th century is considered the *"golden age"* of spanking literature, with the distributions of many spanking novels accompanied by illustrations. However, this golden age came to an end due to the introduction, in Europe, of various censorship laws during the second world war. Recently, the proliferation of the internet has allowed many individuals to get in touch with each other and start spreading material on the subject again. Spanking can be administered with the bare hand, but also tools can be used. The variety of spanking tools is immense, among the most famous we can find:

- Cane
- Paddle
- Slipper
- Wooden spoon
- Carpet beater

Depending on the tool used, the sensation transmitted will be different. For instance, a cane gives a *"stingy"* feeling, a sharp and quick-burning sense mostly felt on the skin. On the other hand, being spanked with a paddle gives a *"thuddy"* sensation that penetrates deeper into the body tissues. Safety is always essential in these types of practices; mainly when you are using spanking tools, it is crucial to avoid striking the tailbone and the hipbones of the receiver.

Spanking is excellent combined with roleplay; for instance, you could try a teacher-student scenario and punish your naughty partner with a ruler. Soft spanking, with the bare hand, can be used during the foreplay or in the most aroused phases of sexual intercourse. Although, I have to admit that I don't mind a good spanking while I'm in doggy style!

6.6 ANAL PLAY & SEX

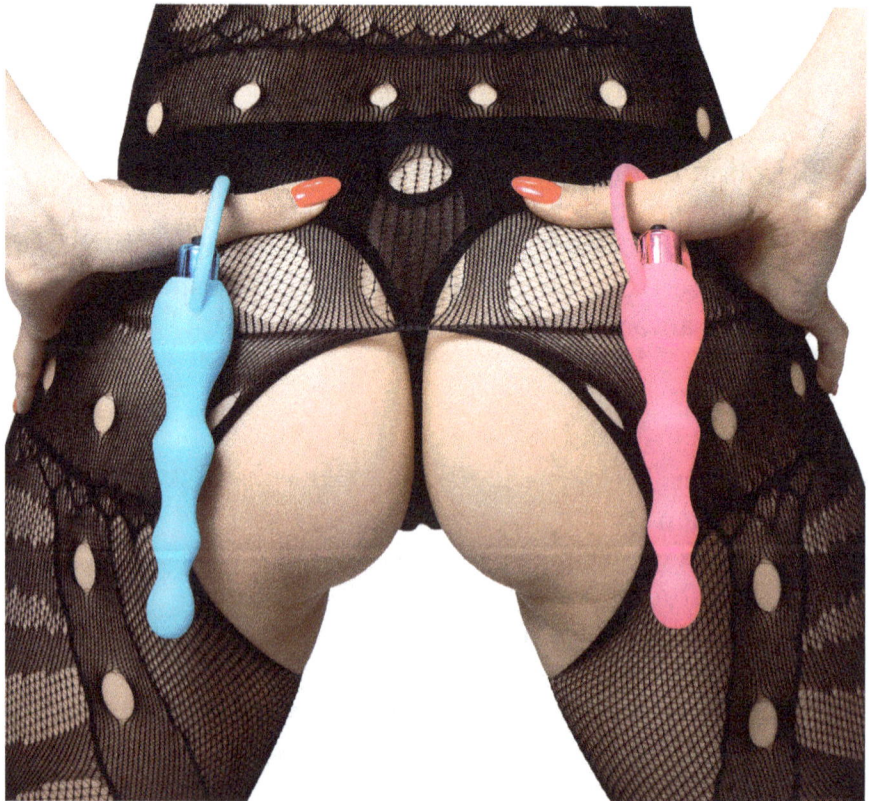

A few years ago, it was much more challenging to talk about anal play and anal sex, while nowadays, you cannot see a comedy show without hearing at least three jokes about anal sex, pegging, and its derivatives. Despite this, the general impression is that there is still a bit of shame to talk about it openly. Well, let me tell you, anal sex is incredible! You do not have to have an anal fetish to take part in anal sex; however, many individuals explicitly get off on butt stuff.

Anal play can go from adding a finger in the ass during penetrative vaginal sex to utilizing butt attachments to having anal sex with a penis or a dildo. In a new report, 37 percent of ladies and 43 percent of men said they had tried anal sex (in which ladies got and men gave). *"The anal opening and canal have a wealth of nerve endings that are primed for pleasure,"* says Caitlin V., MPH, clinical sexologist for Royal. This means that anyone can experience pleasure, sometimes even orgasm, from anal stimulation, regardless of gender or genitals. If you are interested in the topic, I will give you some ideas about the most common practices in this section.

Clean yourself
Before starting anal sex, whether you are a man or a woman, it is recommended to clean up the area to avoid unpleasant inconveniences. A shower or a wet wipe can do the job. In addition, it is advisable to empty the bowels 45 minutes before intercourse.

Use a lot of lube
The critical thing to keep always in your mind is that the anus does not self-lubricate. Therefore, to avoid painful problems, it is advisable to use a good quantity of lubricant. The choice of the type of lubricant depends on what objects you are going to use for penetration.

- Use a **silicone-based lube** if you are playing with fingers or objects made in wood or stainless steel.

- Use a **water-based lube** if you are using a silicone toy.

Get relaxed and in the mood

It is essential to be relaxed before starting any anal play or anal sex activity. The anus is an extremely sensitive area, and in the act of penetration, if the recipient has contracted muscles, there is a risk of causing micro-injuries. Natural ways for relaxing are a warm bath, essential oils, deep breathing, or just playing with yourself. In addition, stimulating your genitals or other erogenous zones and becoming aroused will significantly relax your muscles in the area.

Also, remember to start slowly and gently; you have to give your body time to get used to it.

Anal activities

There are different activities that you could, alone or with your partner.

Anal sex: Well, this is self-explanatory. I suggest starting with doggy style or with the receiver lying on the back. These are the most accessible position and allow for the maximum spread of the area.

Prostate stimulation: Guess what, men G-Spot is the prostate, and it can be reached through anal stimulation. There are specific toys designed to stimulate the prostate on the market, but it can be done with your fingers as well. The important thing is to use a good amount of lube and take it at your own pace. Finding the prostate is not complex; you could do this massage yourself or with the help of your partner.:

- Apply lube.
- Insert the index finger slowly to the first knuckle, to it a couple of times applying lube.

- When you feel the area is well-lubricated, insert up to the second knuckle and repeat the previous steps until you reach the third knuckle.

- Once the finger is comfortably inserted, search for a rounded lump roughly 4 inches inside the rectum and up towards the root of the penis. This is the prostate, and it is extremely sensitive.

- You can massage the prostate in a circular motion or back and forth but gently.

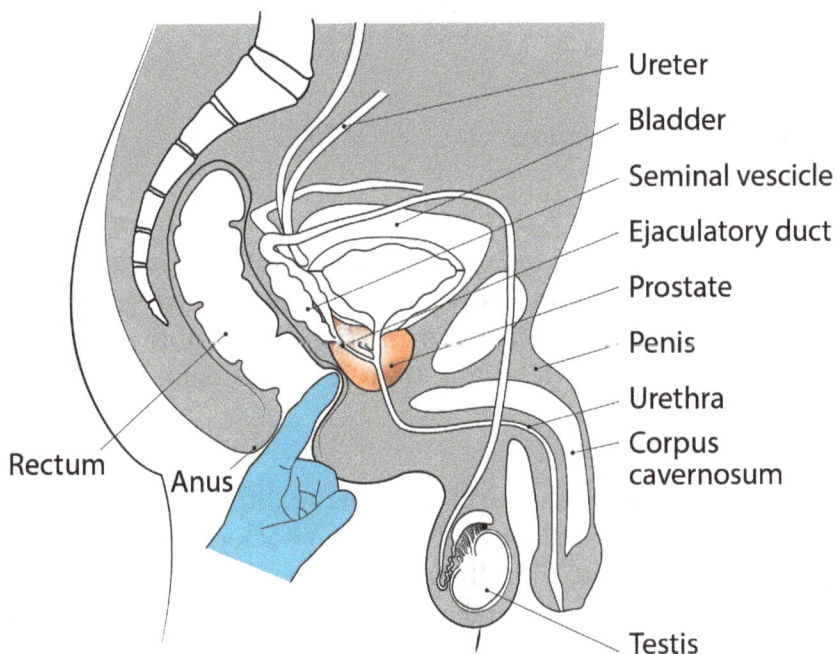

Ureter

Bladder

Seminal vescicle

Ejaculatory duct

Prostate

Penis

Urethra

Corpus cavernosum

Rectum

Anus

Testis

Pegging: This practice is fantastic and gives the woman an incredible sense of power. It consists of penetrating her man with a strap-on dildo. For pegging, a double ending dildo can be used; one side can penetrate the anus while the other is inserted in the vagina. I have tried this practice with my man a few times, and we both loved it. What I can suggest is to start small and with a double-ended dildo. There are strap-ons on the market that do not require any harnesses, but I have personally found hard to use them. I do prefer the harness version, which is much more stable. Also, consider buying one with a vibration function for extra pleasure.

Butt plugs: They can be an excellent addition to your sex life; butt plugs are specifically designed to be inserted into the rectum, even for long periods. These toys are generally smooth and short and can be used during sex by both men and women to provide additional stimulation to the rectum. So if you want to try some light butt stuff and have a different stimulation during sex, butt plugs are what you are looking for.

6.7 Beyond the Bedroom

In the Rain
Have you tried having sex in the shower and enjoyed it? Then, why not trying having sex under a summer shower? Whether you like it or not, you will have another memorable experience, and in my case, a cold, having tried it in October.

In The Bathroom
From the edge of the sink to the side of the shower, the washroom is brimming with perfect spots to push back on when you and your accomplice next get the desire to have sex. Likewise, the shower is ideal for a sensual encounter – all that running water, shower oil, and a lot of snares and edges to grasp – incredible for those couples who appreciate sex in a standing position.

In The Kitchen
The kitchen tabletop is a classic used in numerous movies on the big screen, yet why not try it for yourself at home. There are plenty of positions that adapt perfectly to kitchen surfaces, and this room is accompanied by many interesting objects. For example, you could play with some ice cubes on your partner's body, administer some nice spanking with a spatula or tie your

accomplice to the fridge handles while having sex in a standing position. Every room can be your pleasure room if you use a little creativity.

In The Car

Whenever you and your accomplice are on an excursion, return yourself to those insidious teen years, and stop the vehicle on a peaceful dirt road with no traffic. Then, push back the front seats and jump on top of your accomplice in the driving seat for some sex on the road or move both over the backseats where there will be more space to try various positions.

The Woods

If you both share a love for nature, and you have fun camping in the woods, then why not try here? If you can find a sufficiently isolated place, then you could make a portion of the forest your bedroom. Trees are great to lean against, and they can give you the support to try the most varied positions. Also, you will not have to contain your moans of pleasure if there is no one around.

Under the Stars

Find a place with a good view; it could be a top of a hill, a rooftop, or the bed of a truck. Whatever allows you to see the sky without the light pollution of the city. A starry sky above your head and the person you love next to you is the perfect recipe to create an unforgettable moment. Bring a couple of glasses and some chilled wine with you; this is the ideal scenario for making love and abandoning yourself entirely in your partner's arms.

6.8 CUCKOLDING

Ok, this is not for everyone. However, suppose you are not familiar with Cuckolding. In that case, I think the definition provided by Chris Riotta could help: "the term alludes to when a man or woman has sex with a partner who is already married to someone else. Sometimes, it is out of wedlock, and the experience is essentially just cheating with a fancy term. Other times, it's a fetish in which some married partners enjoy watching their spouse have sex with other partners."

As I said, this is not for everyone, I think I would go crazy to see my man having sex with another woman, but plenty of people find this idea intriguing. Cuckolding can be experienced at different levels, and it is not always necessary to have relationships with another person. Very often, the very idea of betrayal creates a sense of humiliation in the cuckold that is enough to turn him on.

Here some ideas that you might want to try if you are into this.

Go Shopping for your Lover

Bring your partner with you while shopping for your lover; even worse, make your partner pay for everything you will buy. For example, lingerie shopping is perfect. You could try on different underwear and make it clear that you are buying it to arouse someone else. Verbal play in this type of situation is essential; saying things like "I think X will love fucking me in this black underwear" would turn on any cuckold on the face of the earth.

Flirt Openly with Strangers

While your partner is watching, start to flirt with people in bars or lounges. Have your partner find a seat across the room, where they have a nice view of the situation. If the conversation gets a little bit intimate, then you can decide what to do; you might want to go all the way or stop after a few touches and whispers.

Your Cock is Not Big Enough

In this scenario, you want to humiliate your partner, mentioning the size of your (hypothetical?) lovers; for most women, size matters to a degree. Humiliation is a big part of being a cuckold, and being compared to partner lovers is a source of excitement for many of them.

Use Chastity Devices

A common practice during cuckold play is to force the partner to use a chastity device. The basic idea is that you own and manage his orgasms as you please. Who owns the rights to the partner's orgasms is commonly called keyholder since, in most cases, they hold the key to unlock the chastity device. There are chastity devices for both genders on the market, which can also be worn for long periods. However, chastity belts allow you to perform incredibly long and frustrating tease and denial sessions, which can be pushed to the extreme preventing the partner from having an orgasm even for long periods.

Cuckolding and chastity are two vast and complex worlds that would need a book of their own. In this section, I have limited myself to mentioning their existence and providing some basic ideas. If you think these activities are of your interest, I advise you to look for specific texts on the subject; I do not believe I would do justice to these topics in these few lines.

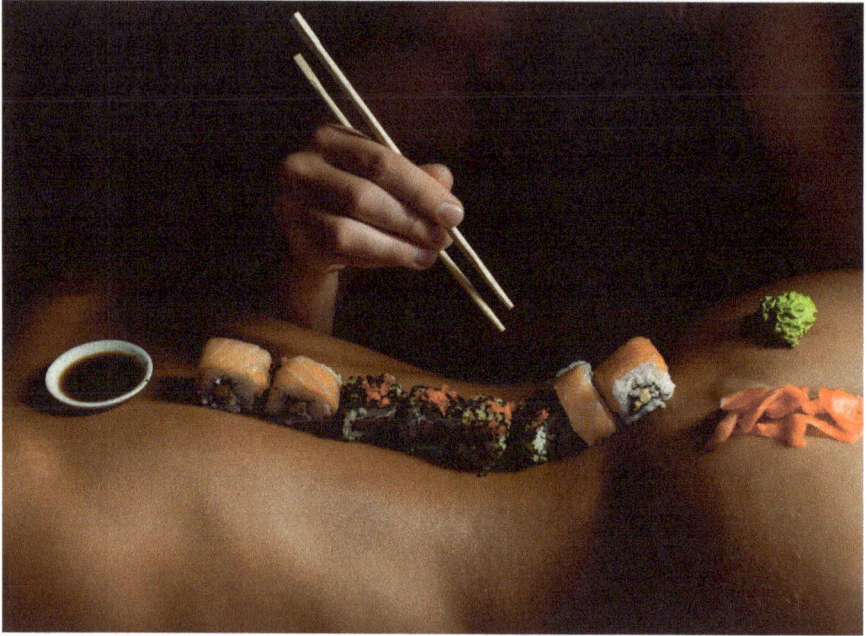

Food can easily be incorporated into your bedroom activities. In addition, many playful ideas can be easily implemented to make sex a lot more interesting.

Cherries

Why not start with a classic? For example, you could challenge your partner to the classic kissing test to see who can tie a cherry stem in a knot with their tongue. Also, cherries are great (especially if cold) to run over your partner's body sensually. Their juice can be drizzled over their erogenous zones and tasted with some tongue play.

Popsicles

Yes, they resemble penises and can be used to show off your blowjob skills. In addition, they are perfect for some foreplay or tease and denial. You could quickly drive your partner crazy at the thought that his penis might be in your mouth instead of the popsicle.

Grapes

Grapes are the perfect fruit if you want to do some roleplay and become queen for one night. Let your partner feed you, one grape at a time, "*Cleopatra style.*" Also, frozen grapes can be used for temperature play. Have your love pluck a frozen grape from its stem and run it over your nipple and other erogenous zones.

Whipped Cream

Yes, I know, it is a little obvious, but I love whipped cream! Spread it on some erogenous zones of your choice and serve an unforgettable dessert to your partner! Penis shafts are fun to decorate with whipped cream, but I suggest not inserting the dessert inside the labia since sugar can cause yeast infections.

Chocolate syrup

If you like whipped cream, then this is the next level. It is a little messier and requires more tongue work to lick it off your lover, but it is also a lot of fun. Also, if you feel creative, you could use it to draw or write messages on your partner's body.

6.10 SENSORY DEPRIVATION

The idea behind sensory deprivation is to limit one or more senses during sex to sharpen the rest. The basic idea is to experience sexual intercourse on another level by amplifying sensations that would not have the same impact in the presence of all the senses.

Sight deprivation

Something as simple as wearing a blindfold or switching off the lights can be remarkably exciting. If you do not see what is about to happen, fear and curiosity will act as amplifiers of the sensations you are experiencing.

Sound-play

Blocking out sounds using wireless headphones can be a powerful weapon. Instead of using white noise, I prefer to pick some music that can better contextualize the moment. For example, if you feel particularly kinky, why not play an audio of people moaning with pleasure.

VR experience

If you have a VR headset, you should try this technique. Have your partner sit in a chair with the headset on and headphones with noise cancellation. Pick porn that your partner likes and show it to them in VR if you have a second screen, even better since you will be able to see what your partner is seeing. Your partner will be almost totally isolated from the outside world, and your goal will be to make the VR experience even more immersive. Stimulate them as you see fit; you can touch his erogenous zones, give them oral sex, or simply let them feel the heat of your body by rubbing on them. The experience will be even more incredible if you contextualize the stimulations with what they see on the screen.

6.11 SEX TOYS

By now on the market, there are dozens of sex toys for the most diverse tastes. Here is a list of the most famous and their functions. I am sure you will find some that will pique your interest.

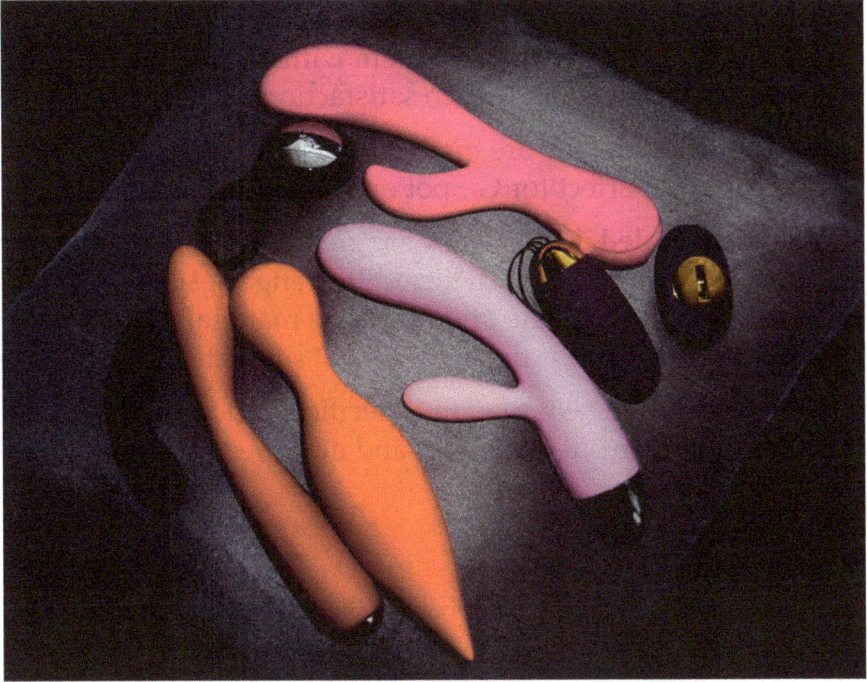

Dildos

Such things are made in different sizes, shapes, and shadings. It ought to be noticed that the male penis, on average 15-18 cm, when dildos, can arrive at 35-40 cm long. Dildos are incredibly versatile and can be an excellent prelude to sex. They can help to get excited and warm up your body before sex. The most common types are:

- **Silicone dildos:** Unlike those in rubber, they cannot cause allergic reactions. They are smooth and firm, perfect for vaginal and rectal activities.

- **Vibrating dildos:** They use a series of sophisticated micromotors to introduce different levels of vibration. They usually cost more, but the incredible additional stimulation justifies the cost.

- **Inflatable dildos:** These dildos are designed to inflate once inserted! They are typically made of flexible latex or rubber, and some can incorporate vibrations functions as well. For example, you can pump up them with air creating a full-up feeling that stretches you to satisfaction.

- **Glass dildos:** They are made of borosilicate glass; the firm material is perfect for G-Spot or prostate stimulation.

- **Double-ended dildos:** They are great for sharing with your partner. They come in an incredible range of sizes, and they are made of bendable and twistable materials. You will be able to try positions that you did not suspect existed before.

- **Anal dildos:** Their shape is specifically designed for anal play. They are often slimmer and designed to stimulate the rectum and the prostate.

Vaginal balls

Kegel balls or *Ben Wa* balls have been used for centuries to increase the strength of pelvic and vagile floor muscles. However, nowadays, they are mainly used for enhancing sexual pleasure; for this reason, they are also called Venus balls or orgasms balls. Vaginal balls are not used in the same way as traditional sex toys; to get the maximum pleasure, you must leave them inside, and they will multiply your fun during masturbation.

Magic wand

This was initially marketed as a general body massager for sore muscles until the '70s when it became famous for its secondary use, one of the best vibrators for clitoral stimulation.

Butt plugs

These are designed to be inserted into the rectum and come in different sizes and sets. Unlike dildos, they are intended to be left inserted even for relatively long periods and can be worn to amplify the sensations resulting from regular sexual activity.

Rabbit vibrators

This is the sex toy no girl should be without! These vibrators are great for clitoral stimulators, and the shaft guarantees intense and extended orgasms. It is also suitable for anal stimulation in case you want to try something different.

6.12 APHRODISIACS

An aphrodisiac is a food or a substance that, when ingested, drives individuals to turn out to be sexually stimulated.
Numerous individuals will utilize these as a fun and coy approach to get them and add their accomplice in the temperament for sex.

Liquor, Marijuana, and Drugs
Cannabis and liquor are the two aphrodisiacs that work by bringing down restraints in the psyche. Suppose you have at any point been affected by both of these. In that case, you may have seen that you felt more secure when it came to stroll over to the bar to converse with that appealing individual you had been looking at or that you were more forward in your sexual advances with your accomplice. This is because these substances brought down your hindrances, which permitted your sexual driving forces to take the driver's seat and persuaded you to do things that you, in any case, would not have because of the expanded sensations of excitement that you were encountering.

Ginseng
Ginseng is a spice that is frequently utilized in Chinese Medicine. In addition, it is extensively used to treat erectile dysfunctions and can prompt more noteworthy degrees of sexual excitement in ladies. It can be ingested in different ways, yet the most well-known route in Asia is ginseng tea.

Pistachio
Pistachio nuts are demonstrated to be an aphrodisiac. These nuts are found in various dishes, both flavorful and sweet, and

can be ingested entirety. Pistachios are used, in some cultures, to cure erectile dysfunction in men as it increases bloodstream. In ladies, it can cause increased sexual excitement. Other than being aphrodisiacs, pistachios have numerous other medical advantages, including weight control and improving heart functionalities.

Saffron

This rare and expensive spice must be collected by hand, and many flowers are required to make just a few grams. Historically, it has been utilized as a solution for tiredness and psychological issues. Nowadays, it has been theorized that this spice can help increase sexual appetite. Saffron is a powerful aphrodisiac, and it is used with individuals who are on antidepressants since it can help balance the diminished sexual drive they cause.

Chocolate

The Aztecs may have been the first on record to draw a link between the cocoa bean and sexual drive. Nowadays, we know that the aphrodisiac qualities of chocolate are due to two substances contains tryptophan and phenylethylamine. So, consuming chocolate can help increase sexual appetite and provide the right amount of energy for a memorable night.

Oysters

It is a widespread belief that oysters are a powerful aphrodisiac. There is no scientific basis to support this theory, but indeed an excellent fish-based dinner can put anyone in the best mood. It is probably not a great idea to play in bed with oysters but organizing a romantic candlelit oyster-based dinner will help to spark the passion.

Honey

Honey has been considered an aphrodisiac for centuries; the very word honeymoon stems from the hope for a sweet marriage. It is known that Hippocrates prescribed honey for sexual vigor, and in an old French tale, receiving a bee sting was like being given a shot of pure aphrodisiac. For these reasons, honey is the symbol of fertility and procreation in many cultures. At the chemical level, honey contains a substance called boron that can contribute to regulating hormone levels. Playing with honey in bed can be messy but sweet (literally).

6.13 EXERCISES TO IMPROVE THE SEXUAL PERFORMANCE

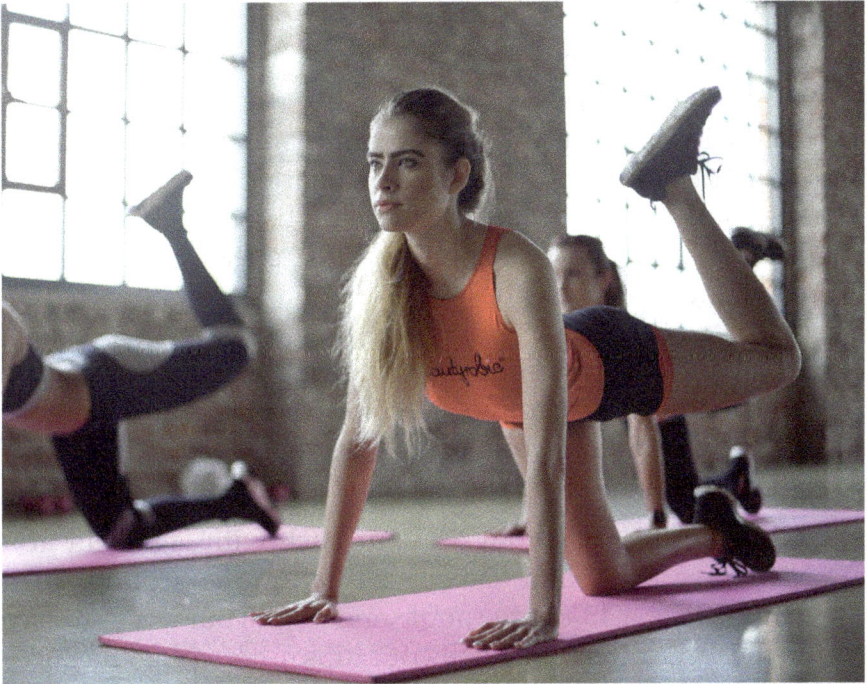

Some may not like hearing it, but an excellent physical condition generally leads to improved quality of sexual intercourse. Without going to extremes, with the stories of people who have had a heart attack while having sex, improving your physical condition can increase the duration and intensity of the performance. Doing physical activity activates specific processes in the body that are similar to those activated during sexual intercourse. We all know that having sex increases sweating, heart activity, and blood flow, just as it would with a running session.

Having sex can be considered physical activity; some studies have calculated that, for each minute, 4.2 calories are burned on average for men and 3.1 for women; the problem is the average duration of sex, which is around 20 minutes. This implies that the total calories burned are not high. For these reasons, it is best to try to burn our calories and get in shape by going to the gym or doing other sports activities.

20 Minutes Training

The following routine does not require any gym equipment, and it should take only 20minutes. I started doing it twice a week, and after a month, I have already begun to see the first results! Set a timer to 20 minutes and repeat the following exercises until the timer goes off.

- **Planks:** Plant your forearms on the floor with elbows below your shoulders. Ground toes into the floor and squeeze glutes to stabilize your body. Put your head in line with your back. Hold the position for 30 seconds.

- **Glute bridge:** Start flat on your back with legs bent at a 90-degree angle and feet placed flat on the ground. Turn your toes at a 45-degree angle and align your knees to face in the same direction. Push your hips up, keeping the knees over your toes throughout the entire movement. Let your hips sink back and repeat (this counts as one repetition). Perform three sets of 15 repetitions.

- **Jump squat:** Stand with your feet shoulder-width apart. Start by doing a regular squat, then engage your core and jump up. When you land, lower your body back into a squat position to complete one repetition. Do two sets of 10 repetitions.

- **Kegels:** Ensure that your bladder is empty, then sit down.

Tighten your pelvic floor muscles. Hold tight and count 3 to 5 seconds. Next, relax the muscles and count 3 to 5 seconds. Perform two sets of 10 repetitions.

- **Pushups:** Start in a high plank position with your palms flat. Bend your elbows and lower your chest to the floor. Push through the palms of your hands to straighten your arms. This counts as one reap. Perform three sets of 8 repetitions.

Try Yoga

Yoga is the discipline par excellence to improve your sexual performance; not only can it be used as stress relief, but it increases the flexibility of the body, coordination and strengthens the core muscles Yoga. Suppose you are a particularly emotional or stressed person. In that case, you will find immense benefits in practicing yoga since it reduces cortisol levels, one of the leading causes of stress.

"Yoga teaches you how to listen to your body and how to control your mind," says Lauren Zoeller, a certified yoga instructor and Whole Living Life Coach based in Nashville, Tennessee. *"These two practices combined can bring your insight on what you like and dislike, leading you to communicate better what is best to your partner."*

If you want to try Yoga, I suggest looking for a course close to home so you can learn the basics from a professional.
I will list here the yoga positions that, in my experience, have the most significant impact in terms of stress relief and fitness improvement. I would suggest that you perform them supervised by a professional so that you can learn the correct execution of each position.

1. Marjaryasana / Bitilasana

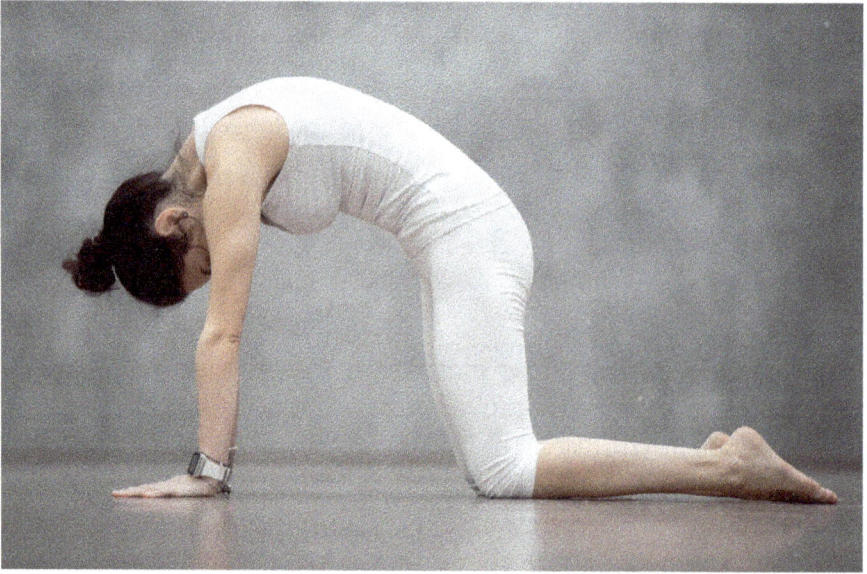

This is a gentle flow between two positions that mainly involves the back muscles and the spine. The starting position is on hands and knees with knees under the hips and hands under the shoulders, head in a neutral position. To move into *Bitilasana*, inhale and drop your belly towards the mat. Gaze up towards the sky, lifting chin and chest. Open your shoulders and relax, feeling the stretch on the spine. To transition into *Marjaryasana*, exhale and draw your belly to your spine while rounding the back towards the sky. Release your head towards the floor. Repeat the cycle up to 20 times.

2. Setu Bandha Sarvangasana

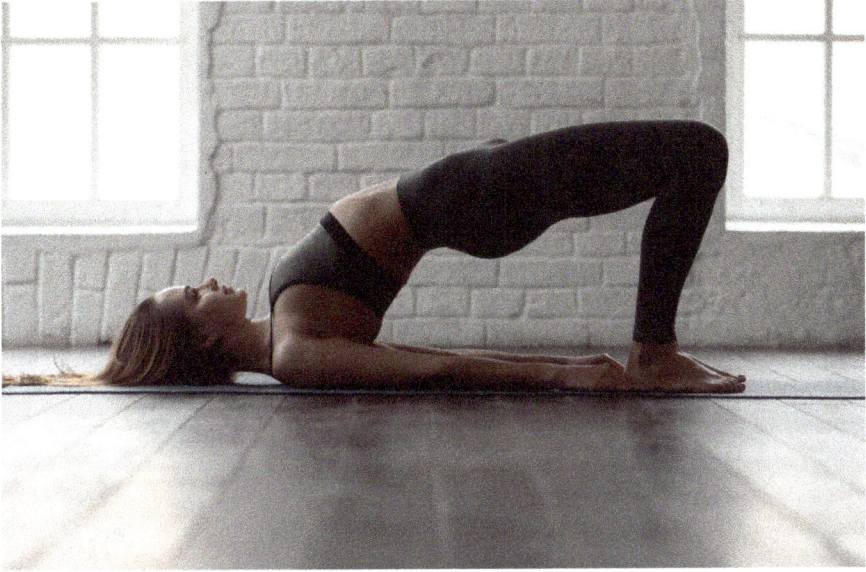

Lie on your back with knees bent and feet firmly on the floor. Place your arms on either side of your body with your palms facing down. Exhale as you lift your hips towards the sky while pressing both feet and arms into the floor. Roll your shoulders back. The only parts in contact with the floor must be your arms, feet, head, and upper back.

3. ANANDA BALASANA

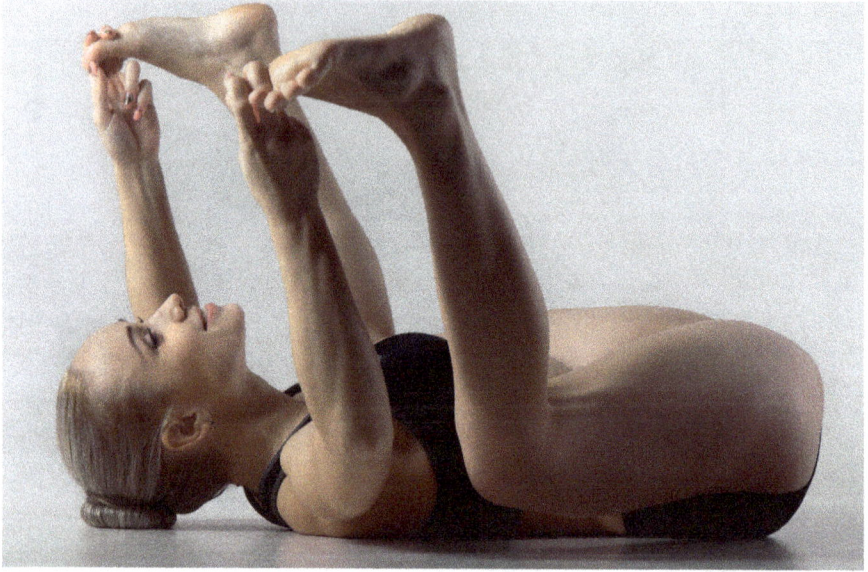

Lie on your back, and while exhaling, bend your knees into your belly. Inhale and grip your feet or toes with your hands. Open your knees slightly wider than your torso and bring them up toward your armpits. Be sure that each ankle is positioned over the knee.

4. Child's Pose – Balasana

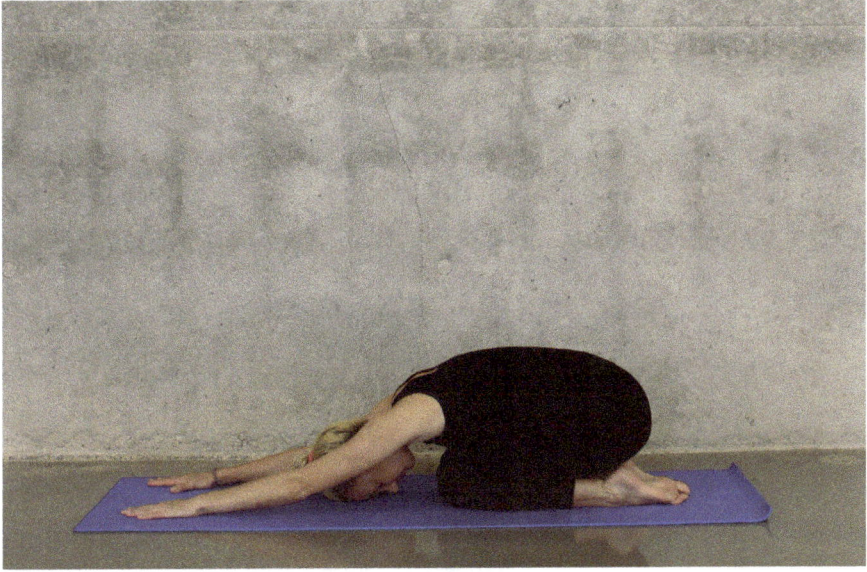

Come to your hands and knees on the mat. Slightly spread your knees and keep the top of your feet on the floor. Bend, bringing your forehead to the floor. It is essential to relax your spine, shoulders, and jaw. Stay as long as you like, feeling the nice stretch on your spine.

5. SAVASANA

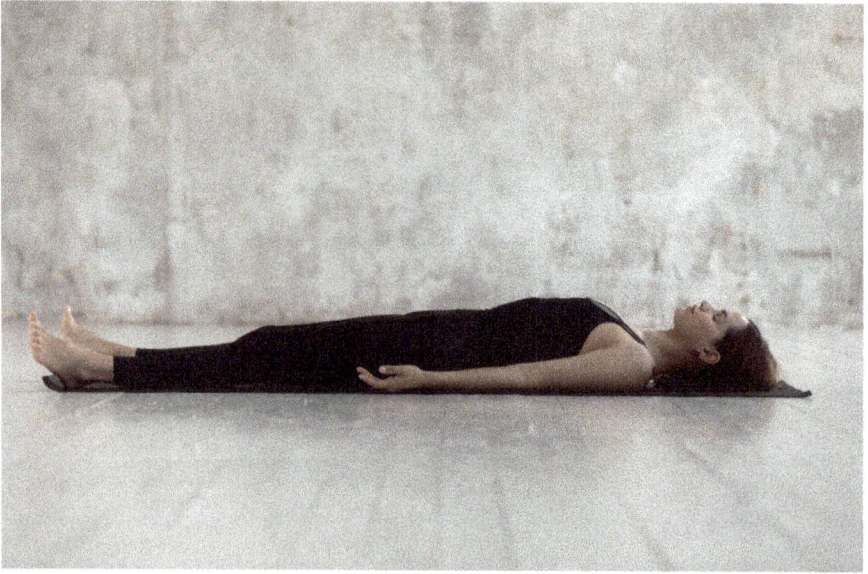

Lie on your back with legs and arms straight, palms facing upward. Stay as long as you like focusing on your breathing.

While some yoga poses can immediately improve your sex life, the most significant change will always reduce your stress. Not only does this provide a whole host of benefits, but it also allows you to relax and enjoy sex, which makes it even better.

The Invisible Chair Exercise

This exercise is perfect for those with little time and no equipment. To perform "the invisible chair," put your back flat against a wall with your hands open on the surface of the wall. Next, bring your legs forward and flex your knees until you reach a position where you are sitting supported only by the wall. Once this is done, try to hold the position as long as possible. Repeat for at least three times with 60 seconds of rest between each attempt. This exercise is a simple, easy and effective way to work your core and lower body, so grab a wall and relax in your "Invisible Chair"!

Conclusion

I wrote this book with the idea of sharing what I have learned from my experiences around the world and my passion for Indian culture.I hope, in this manuscript, you found what you were looking for, be it a new position, some new ideas, or topics to start a conversation with your partner to deepen your relationship. As you have learned by now, the Kama Sutra is not just a series of sexual positions; it is a way of approaching a relationship, love, and life in general. Moreover, the original text consisted of more than 500 pages, some difficult to interpret, others totally out of context for modern times. For these reasons, I have not tried to provide my readers with an exact copy of the original work. I tried instead to extract the parts that, in my opinion, are most relevant in modern society, and I have mixed them with some suggestions and ideas from my personal experience. I hope the result was exciting and that I was able to convey the fundamental principles of the Kama Sutra to you.

If there is one thing that I mainly wanted to convey to you, it is the idea that there is no right or wrong in making love. Two or more people are free to experience everything they want to try together and thus seek new incredible sensations. It is essential to cultivate love and try new experiences, especially in relationships that we believe have been solid and have lasted for many years. This allows us to continue to renew the flame of passion and live a whole and happy life.

TANTRIC SEX
Guide for Couples

Explore the Path of Sacred Sex to Reach the Ultimate Pleasure.
Spice Up Your Sex Life Through Meditation, Breathing, and
Illustrated Tantra Sex Positions

SAMANTHA MANDALA

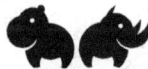

IPPOCERONTE
publishing

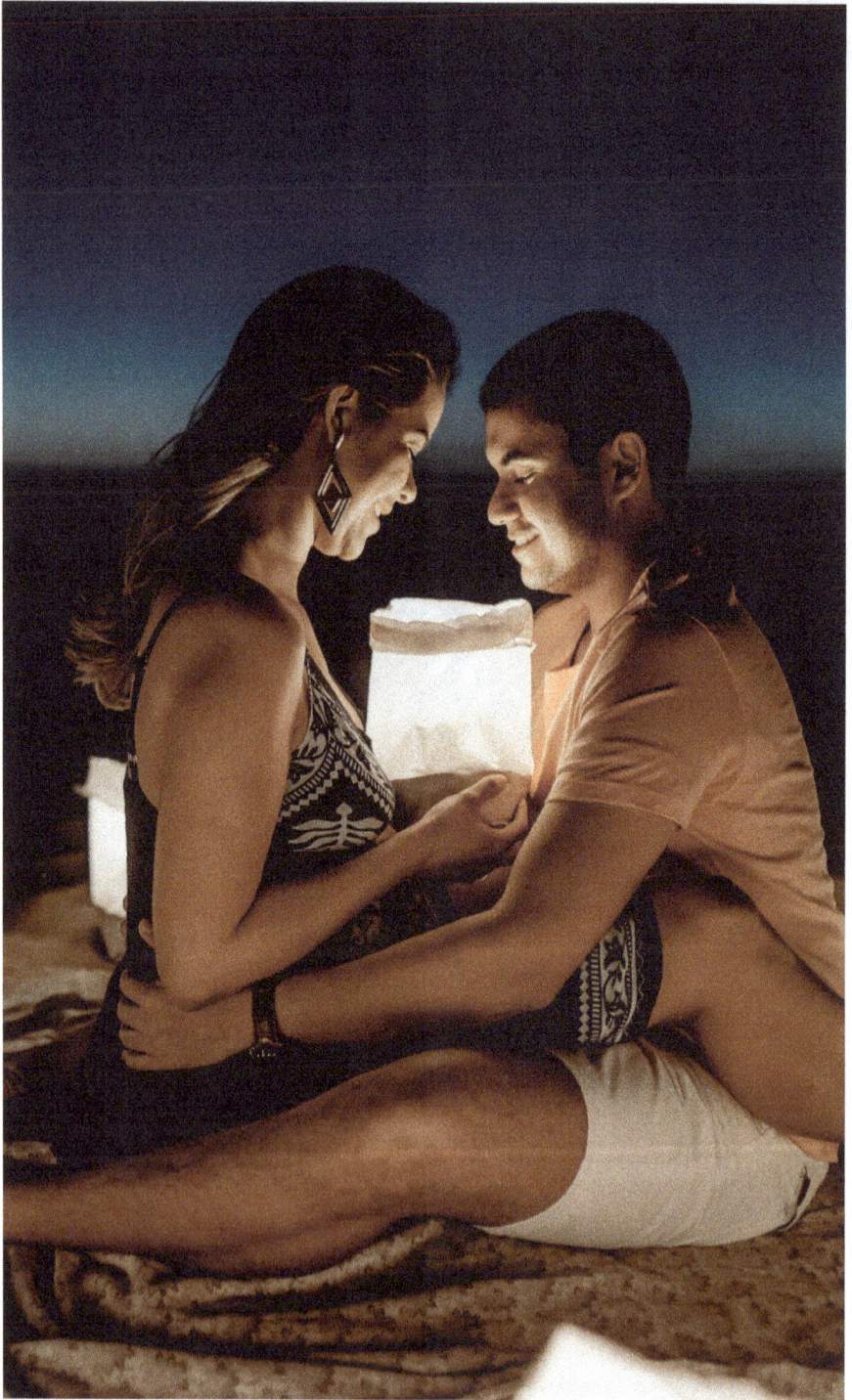

Introduction

We learn about sex in school and build it in our imagination through stories, movies, novels, and commercials. But the intercourse showed by the media is often an exaggeration: the whole circumstances are often extreme but romantic, and the act of sex itself is like a take-breath-away experience imagined with firecrackers and flashes.

This visualization of sex may cause pressure in ordinary life, and real people may want to perform like the characters they see in those movies. This sort of portrayal has set in individuals' psyches significantly elevated requirements that are hard to accomplish in reality, particularly from young couples who need insight.

When the experience isn't just about as high as envisioned, individuals may feel disappointed and lose self-assurance. Likewise, they may believe that the entire relationship has lost its enthusiasm and is near the precarious edge of self-destructing.

Simultaneously, sex sometimes is a level battleground. We might be searching for sexual intimacy at the core of our being, yet in addition, we take incredible consideration to evade it. Maybe we need to be contacted with our entire heart yet dread our shortcomings. We may take longer to recover lost energy yet have failed to remember how to light the fire.

From what I can see, there is a significant misreading of sex inside the western culture because the sexual education given to us since our best age is limited to only physical and biological activity. Sex could be much more than an instinct that pushes creatures to procreate, and it's also much more than an activity for "having a great time." Sex can be an instrument to explore our body and our way to pleasure, and it's also the best venture to connect with our partner.

In some east cultures, lovemaking is a ritual that deals not only with the physical world but also with the spiritual one. And this is what we call Tantra.

Tantra is not the mere act of sex made to please ourselves and our partner. Instead, it's a whole journey that carries humans close to the divinities using the "dance" of our bodies.

Whatever you are looking for a spiritual journey or just for suggestions to get the best experience from the act of love, Tantra can help you explore yourself and to learn more about pleasure and discover what you like. Learning about Tantra is also the best way to improve the relationship between couples since this discipline teaches the path to knowledge through the connection with a partner.

The way of thinking of Tantra shows us how to recuperate our sexual intimacy. Also, with this ancient practice, we can discover new sensual delights and change simple snapshots of sexual pleasure into the existence of sexual ecstasy.

When everyday stress, fears, and interruptions compromise relationships, Tantra practice shows us how to open our hearts, get in touch with our emotions and sexuality.

With everything on the planet today being rushed, hurried,

and loaded with pressure, we don't invest sufficient energy appreciating the pleasure. Easy-going sex and quick ones have supplanted intimacy and love, and it appears that nobody has "the time" any longer to live sex how it was intended to.

Sex is not only a physical act; it is two souls meeting up to make a sexual encounter that rises above the actual limits. Tantric sex is an action where couples participate in different sexually and sincerely fulfilling encounters to help blend their spirits.

The tantric sex approach takes things gradually, appreciating each experience and getting a charge out of it. It's not tied in with achieving an orgasm, yet it teaches to enjoying the intimacy you share with your accomplice. Sex shouldn't be an exhibition that simply makes a cursory effort. Where's the association, the love, the intimacy, and the uncommon bond that is possibly divided among lovers when it doesn't convert into your sex life? Lovemaking is far beyond the actual demonstration of sex; it is about creating a bond with your partner.

I know there are many books regarding this matter, and I would like to thank you for your trust in choosing this one! I decided to write this book to share my knowledge about this fascinating topic that opened my mind to new experiences. Like many, I had an ordinary life, spending my life between job, family, and friends. Eventually, I started to lose enthusiasm; even sex couldn't cheer me up. It was when sharing these feelings with one of my friends that he introduced me to Tantra. In the beginning, it was just a game, but I soon realized that our encounters didn't end in bed, but they were bringing benefits into my everyday life. To be specific, my life wasn't changing; I was the one that was seeing things differently because I slowly started to open myself to this world.

Sometimes we need a spark to change our life. Tantra was my spark. It helped me light my everyday routine, find meaning in my existence, and enjoy every pleasure fully.

This book takes the reader on a steady restorative excursion, clarifying the interconnectivity of the activities of your brain, soul, body, climate, and feelings to investigate with your accomplice. Whenever utilized effectively, it can get a special proclivity and put some extra spice in your relationship. Similar to yoga, it plans to locate the correct equilibrium and importance throughout everyday life.

~ CHAPTER 1 ~

Tantra, Meaning and Origins

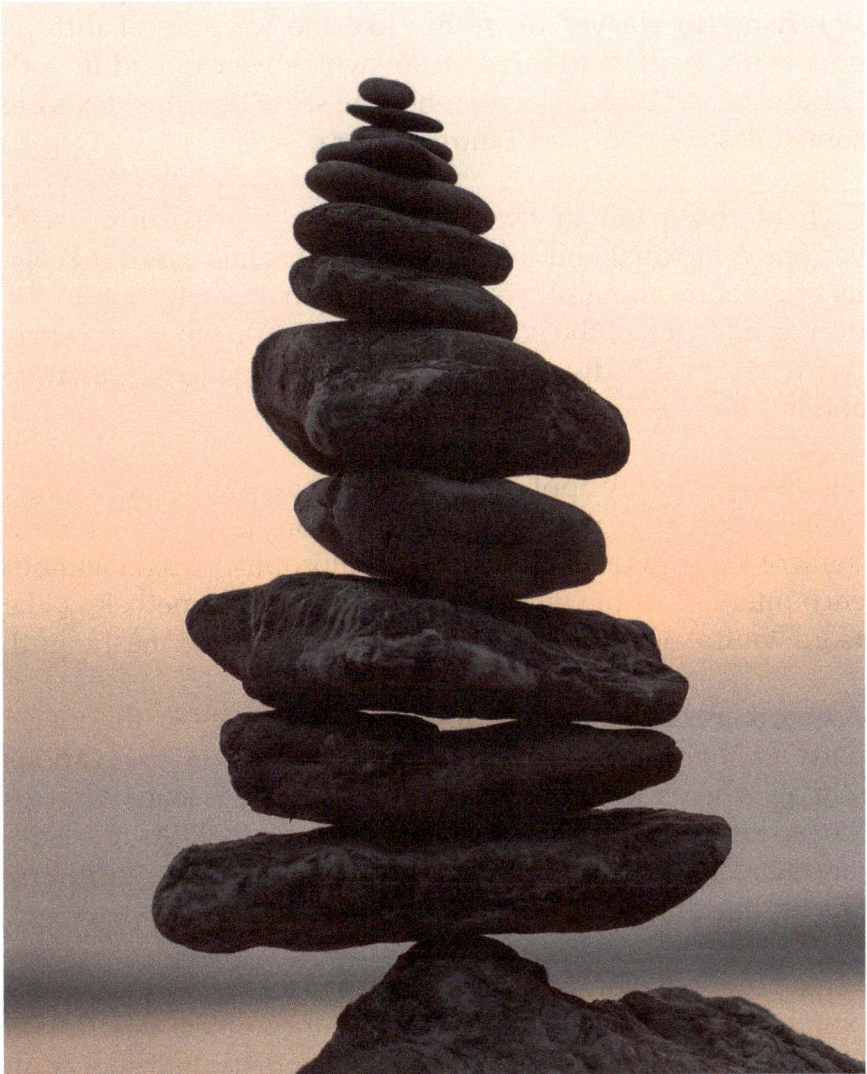

1.1 What is Tantra?

Tantra is a way of thinking that arose in India around the 6th century; it has been connected to progressive influxes of progressive ideas, from its initial change of Hinduism and Buddhism to the Indian battle for autonomy and the ascent of 1960s nonconformity.

The Sanskrit word 'Tantra' comes from the verbal root *tan*, signifying 'to weave,' or 'form,' like the warping of threads on a loom. It refers to sacred texts, which we can find in both Hinduism and Buddhist religions. The same Buddhist texts are sometimes referred to as Tantra or sutra.

Each of those Indian texts applies the word 'Tantra' with various contextual and interpretations. In some cases, it keeps its original meaning of 'wave,' 'warp,' 'loom,' referring to the deep connection of the body and the spirit. On other occasions, this word means 'discipline,' 'rituals and practices,' 'essence,' and in some cases even 'doctrine' and 'science.'

Because of so many applications, Tantra has always had a broad range of meanings and teachings. Therefore, it is not possible to think of Tantra as a single practice, philosophy, or path without encountering people who disagree with you. Nonetheless, the word 'tantra' does refer to something coherent and meaningful.

Asana, mantra, pranayama, reflection, and rituals are the crucial parts of Tantra. These components blended in the various schools where each school varies from the others since it moves the accentuation on some element or another. As a result, tantrism significantly influenced many religions, including Shavis, Buddhism, Vaishnavism, and Jainism.

Some people see Tantra as a kind of "Yoga for sex," which, in my opinion, it would be a superficial and incomplete description by far. Regardless, the part of sex in this discipline shows up only occasionally in the sacred texts.

Other people would rather see it as a religion, which still won't be correct, even if the Tantric symbology and practices have emerged throughout history in many religions and cultures. Tantra may depend on mystical ideas, but it leads to an elevation of the spirit only through the exploration of the human body.

So, forgive me if my definition of Tantra doesn't cover all the meanings acquired in centuries through religious practice and cultural influence over different territories. Probably a whole book won't be enough to cover the meaning of this discipline in all its parts, but for sure, you'll get a better understanding going through this book. For now, consider Tantra as an experience that allows you to explore yourself with your body. You can see it as a journey that will help you to find pleasure in your everyday life.

Thinking about Buddhism, I can even say that, if done correctly, Tantra may even help you to reach the illumination. For example, one of the primary objectives of Buddhism is to overcome desire because it leads to a path of frustration and despair since humans can't be fully satisfied.

The ideal approach to accomplish this is to experience the passion and train it so we would be able to control it. Therefore, whenever utilized accurately, Tantra could show individuals the pathway to accomplish enlightenment.

In some cultures, people believe that some monks or gurus managed to achieve empowerment from this discipline. Like a healthy body and long life, without mentioning a profound elevation of the spirit.

Without a doubt, the tantric methodology assists with mitigating the pressure of the couple. Furthermore, it will give the correct guidance to forget about the "execution tension" and provide an alternative practice where you can discover your pleasure alongside your partner.

1.2 TANTRA TEXTS

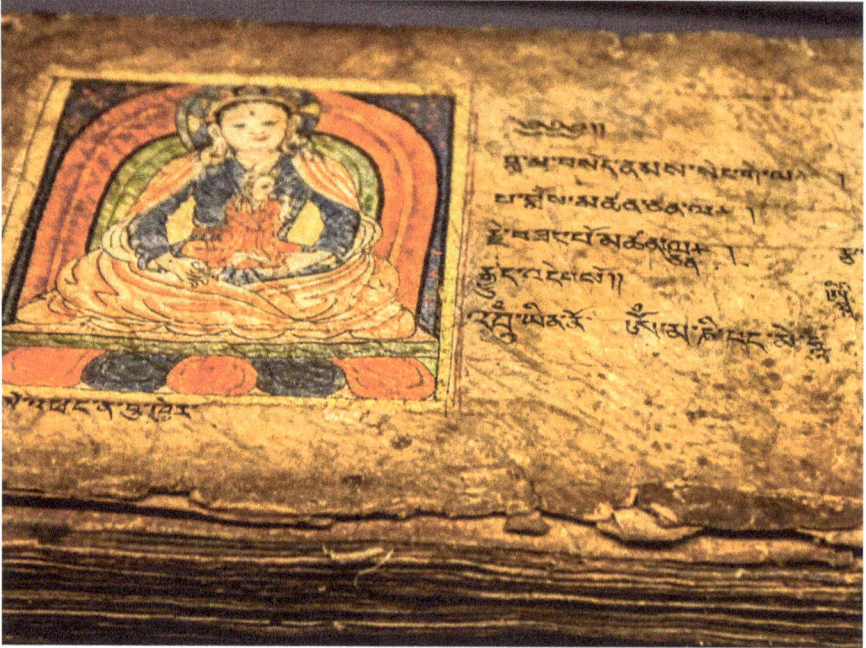

Two primary ancient texts inspired Indian philosophy: Vedas and Tantras. Composed in Sanskrit, the texts constitute the oldest layer of Sanskrit literature and the oldest scriptures of Hinduism. There is still a considerable debate on which one came first, but it is clear that they were born a long time before their transcription as they were initially passed orally.

Even if those two sacred texts aim to reach illumination, they have some disagreement on the approach to apply for the enlightenment. Still, the differences between the two are so minor that sometimes people confuse one with the other.

To see the differences between the two, we should get deep into the details. Still, we can summarize by saying that Tantra exalts individual power and recommended practice, while Vedas gives more authority to collective energy based on rituals in groups. Many people think that the present day of spiritual practices in India is based on Vedas. But in reality, a majority of the rituals and practices are based on Tantra and partly on Vedas.

There are two categories of these sacred texts: Agama and Nigama. Vedas literature is referred to as Nigama and is understood as the highest truth, describing the origin of creation itself. Agamic texts were written much later than Vedas, and the meaning of Agama is "that which has come." The Agamas neither accept nor reject the Vedas, but they use the knowledge revealed in Nigama for appropriate practices.

There are three types of Agamas:

1. Vaishnava Agamas – worship and regard Vishnu as the supreme
2. Shaiva Agamas – worship and regard Shiva as the supreme
3. Shakta Agamas – worship and regard Divine Mother (Shakti) as the supreme

Those texts are the transposition of divine dialogues as the gods themselves wrote them. In particular, the divines Shiva and Shakti or their emanations talking in-person in the sutras, as a conversation between husband and wife where one is asking questions and the other is teaching, as a relationship between student and teacher.

Technically, talking about tantras, we refer to the Shakta Agamas, where the Goddess Shakti has the teacher's role and reveals the knowledge of the creation to the God Shiva.

Tantric texts are written in aphorisms to express complex and ideological concepts that are subjected to different interpretations. This literature has mostly more than one reading and can be experienced at varying levels of intuition. Thus, the same text may be confusing or illuminating, depending on the reader's level of experience.

Today we can count more than 500 existing Tantras, but many of them have not been translated from Sanskrit. We believe that initially, there were more than 14000 volumes and that most of them have been lost over time.

Even if each text is open to different interpretations, it cannot be said that the tantric texts contradict each other; they just give importance to various aspects than others.

1.3 FROM THE ORIGIN TO TODAY

There have been various attempts to determine the origin of Tantra. According to some historians, the first appearance of the tantric practice in the first sacred text is dated around 600 CE. However, some indications show that Tantra may have started its journey from the Bronze Age, around 2000 BC. In this period, the civilization populating the Indus Valley Region was the Harappan from Harappa, the first urban center discovered by archeologists in this territory. This culture was probably the first to build at least one bathroom in their homes, something unheard of for the other civilizations in the same era. They also made a swimming pool in the heart of their capital Mohenjo-Daro, instead of using it as a center for governance and commerce.

Another peculiarity of this civilization is the privileged role that women kept in both society and religion. Statues and items picturing a female figure with open arms and legs spread apart were found in many sanctuaries and buildings. These representations are showing the woman as the mother goddess offering herself to adoration.

It is believed that the woman was the center of the Tantra culture, and for this reason, ladies are allowed to teach the tantra dogma. At the same time, in other religions, like Hinduism, female teachers were forbidden.

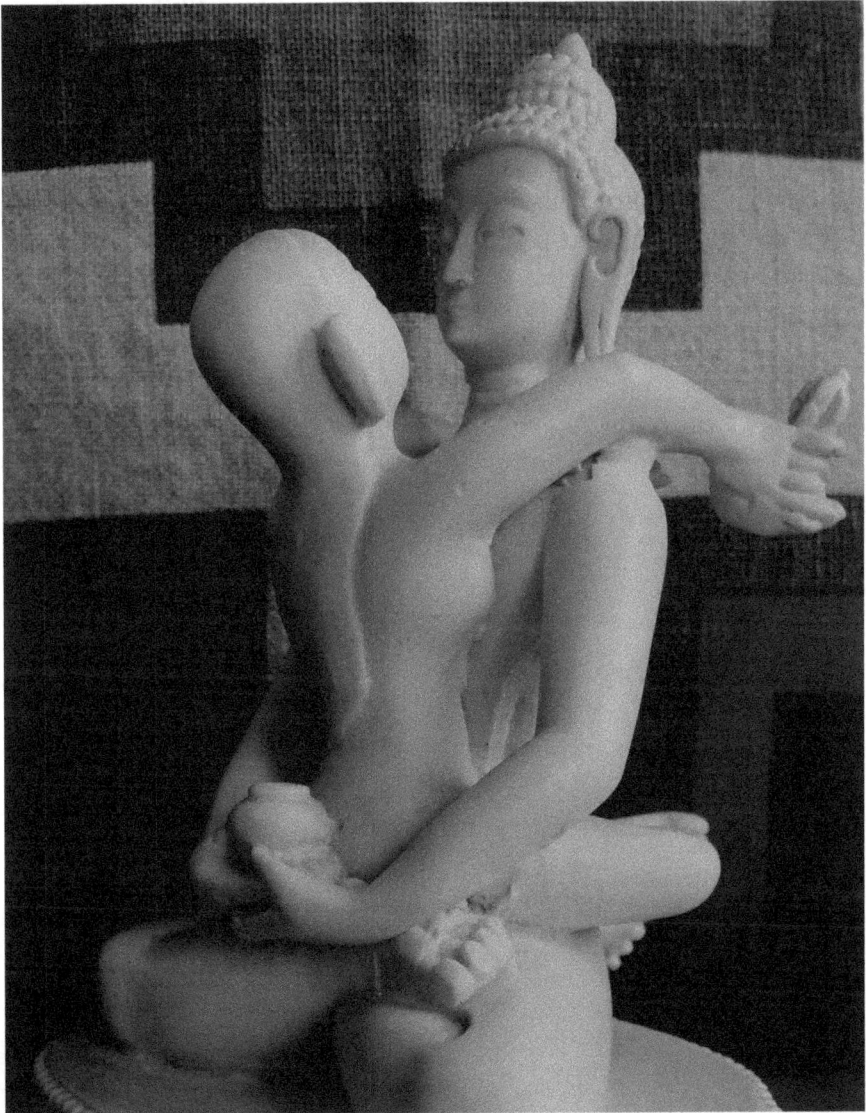

Talking about Tantra, there are two different paths that its practitioners describe: *Dakshinachara* and *Vamachara*.

Dakshinachara is translated as Right-Hand Path and is also known as *white Tantra*. It consists of the traditional practices where enlightenment is reached through asceticism and meditation. White Tantra is an esoteric female-focused tradition, which emphasizes meditation over other practices. The goal of the right path is not to get closer to a deity or achieve liberation from life or death; instead, practitioners focus on their individual journey by uncovering and purifying the mind. White tantric practitioners typically work within four categories: Wisdom Practice, Magical Practice, Mental Practice, and Emotional Practice. Hinduism, Tibetan Buddhism, Kundalini, and Kriya yoga are right-handed paths, all of which follow the traditional tantric practices described.

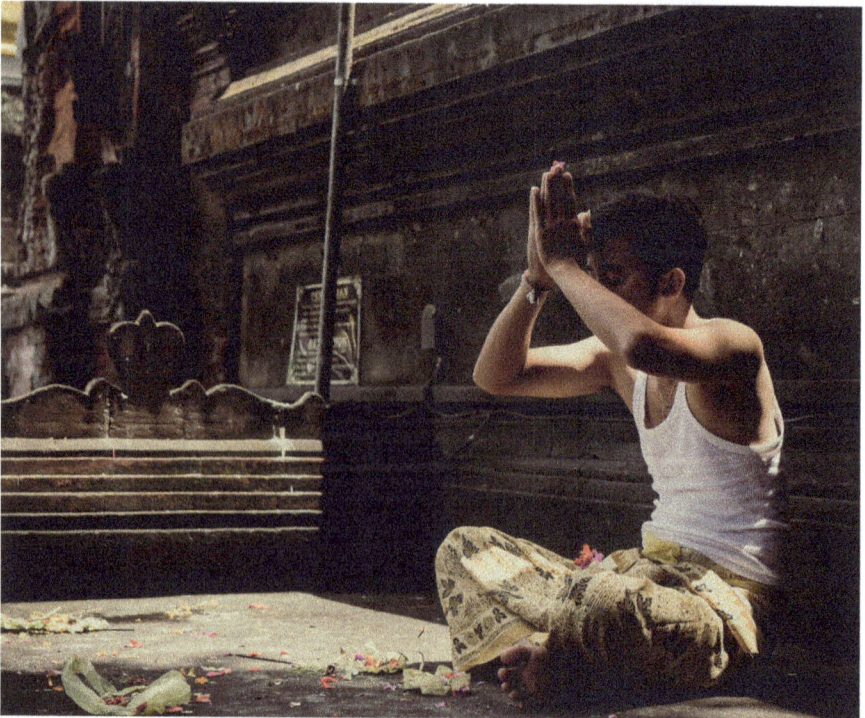

Vamachara is instead the Left-Hand Path, also known as *red Tantra*, and it includes ritual practices in contrast with the white Tantra. Vamachara is attached to materiality and sexual instincts, and this path ritual sex, alcohol, and other intoxications are allowed. It is based on the belief that sexuality can be used in a spiritual and ritualistic way to achieve union with the Divine. Devotees of red Tantra believe that this union can be achieved with any human of any gender. Sexual energy is an element shared with boths the paths but used for different purposes. The final goal of red tantra is to create a profound connection with the partner, while the white path is mostly a solitary journey. Both the paths can bring the *Moksha* (literally 'liberation' or 'nirvana'), but the Vamachara is mainly considered the fastest path.

The alleged "right hand" and "left hand" ways are unmistakably recognized. In the "right hand" path, the male and female divinities becoming one unity is considered an analogy at an energy level. In contrast, the "left hand" methods apply this allegoric image to the physical world.

Subsequently begins *maithuna* - the mysterious custom of love - which isn't a focal practice, although Tantra is today usually connected to it. On the opposite, *maithuna* is viewed as one of the most important and last stages that the yogi should confront because lone genuine yogis can stand to rehearse it as a contemplation method.

1.4 What is Neotantra?

The terminology 'Tantra' arrived in the West in conjunction with the sexual liberation of the 60s and 70s, and women's emancipation helped this teaching spread in America.

Neotantra is a recent and western form of Tantra that has been around for over 150 years. It does take inspiration from Hindu and

Buddhist ideas, but instead of focusing on reaching enlightenment, it pays attention primarily to sex and having a better orgasm. Neotantra is definitely a path inspired by Tantra, even if the two practices have different bases. The strong contrasts between them are: Neotantra depends on present-day books rather than old sacred writings and doesn't need a master for inception. In traditional Indian and Tibetan Tantra, a pioneer (alluded to as a *guru parampara*) is proclaimed as having the most extreme need for spiritual movement. Neotantrics fervently debate this, enticing the idea that anybody anxious to communicate sexually may start on their tantric way.

In contemporary occasions, the most well-known misconception is the qualification among Tantra and tantric sex. Tantra's derivation signifies 'the weaving and development of energy,' yet Tantra itself doesn't include sex by any means as opposed to mainstream thinking. Instead, it's teaching about the union of the manly and ladylike energy that can be accomplished through meditation and breathing procedures.

Its inceptions have been followed in the conventional writings of Hinduism, Buddhism, and other Asian convictions where sexual investigation has frequently been illegal, especially for ladies.

Tantric sex is the point at which these teachings are applied in the room. The matter becomes to develop a more private association among accomplices and a woven association with the Divine. The training isn't 'objective orientated,' yet somewhat a type of love looking to keep its members present all through. While tantric ecstasy and accomplishing the big O may end up happening simultaneously, they are unquestionably not a similar accomplishment.

When most people, especially in Western countries, talk about Tantra these days, they are actually talking about Neotantra. It is likewise intriguing to note that from the mid-late 20th century, as India was fighting for autonomy and finding new support over their public personality, Neotantra turned into a word habitually used to give India attention and merit, spread especially among the Western crowds.

While in 2018, Tantra got inseparable from "spiritual sex" and "holy sexuality," these semantics are dug in undeniably more unpredictable verifiable convictions. Similarly, as with most components of history notwithstanding, mindfulness and appreciation are vital.

Neaotranta is an adapted version of Tantra for the Occidentals, but it does help to spread some of the Eastern values into the Western world.

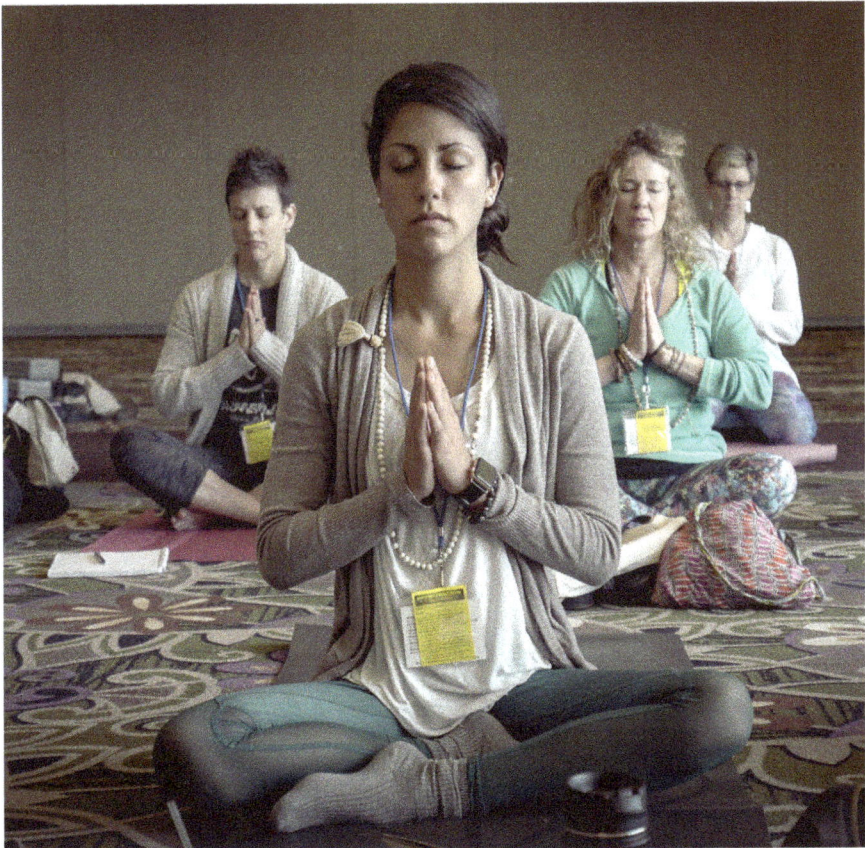

CHAPTER 2

Tantra and Spirituality

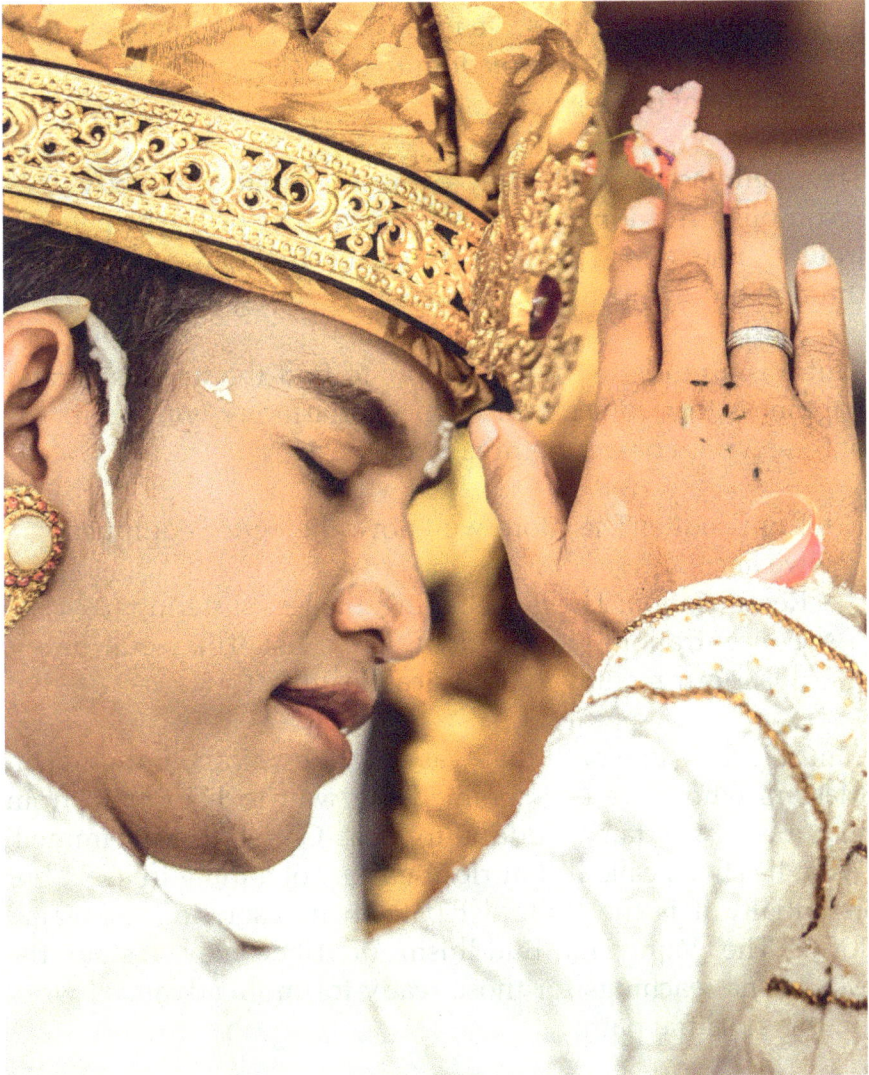

2.1 TANTRA AND THE WAY OF LIBERATION

Tantra is a spiritual way and a lifestyle. It's an individual act of freedom. The act of Tantra frees you up to a spiritual encounter and to understanding the human body and natural life as tangible signs of divine energy. Sexual energy can be an incredible way to spiritual advancement. Life can be incorporated and celebrated on the way to illumination. The Tantric conviction that encountering sexual fervor is a sample of cosmic energy is a significant and progressive idea, as pertinent today as before. Tantra is the method of freedom that opens up to the genuine articulation of oneself.

The Guhyasamaja Tantra expresses that: "nobody can accomplish freedom on the off chance that he participates in troublesome and torturing practices; freedom is reachable through the cognizant satisfaction, everything being equal."

Tantra is a guide that teaches how to find the fulfillment and happiness that comes from being in harmony with your true nature. A path based on three principles:

- Knowledge: The more we know, the better equipped we are.
- Renunciation: The less clinging, the less suffering.
- Concentration: Hold it tight, like a fist. The result of this is our mental and physical health.

Tantra is the same path that was taught by all the Enlightened Masters who have ever pointed the way to liberation, from the time of Gautama Buddha to Jesus Christ, to Mohammed. What has been called "Tantric Yoga" is not a thing in itself, but essentially it is the Buddhist path in its esoteric (Vajrayana) form. The Vajrayana Buddhism of Tibet may restate the Mahayana teachings for those ready for more advanced work on this spiritual path.

Tantra is an ancient yogic practice that helps one achieve a deep meditative consciousness and personal transformation. It can also be used to transform relationships, both with oneself and with a partner.

Tantric practices are based on the fundamental understanding that sexuality is much more than the act of intercourse or genital stimulation. Instead, it is an exchange of energy between two people on all levels: spiritual, emotional, intellectual, and physical. Furthermore, Tantra teaches that this energy can be transmitted through touch to create ecstatic feelings of pleasure for both partners.

Tantra can revitalize even the most "tired" relationships and add new life to sexual expression when practiced regularly. Tantra can also overcome performance anxiety in new or established relationships by focusing on the physical sensations.

Tantric practices can be incorporated into any relationship – married, single, straight or gay. However, the benefits of practicing Tantra are most profound in long-term committed relationships because these are the relationships that have time to evolve and sustain themselves on all levels.

The effects of Tantra are most powerful if both partners practice. However, if one of the partners is not open to practicing Tantra, the benefits can still be significant for the other, especially for women.

2.2 THE SEVEN CHAKRAS

"When your chakras are balanced, you can experience clarity, access power, and feel more joyful, fearless, and free"
Jesse Lucier (2015).

If you dive into Tantra or any spiritual practice coming from the East, you'll face how mind and body are balanced together through masses of energy called chakras.

A chakra is a spinning wheel of energy. When it's spinning fast and in balance with other chakras, you're living in the present moment. But when your chakras get out of whack, life can start to feel constrained and heavy.

Those energy centers interact with the human body by numerous fibers, channels, and energy pathways. They're like the veins of a leaf: every leaf has many veins, but together they all stem from the same trunk. The power lies in how everything works together as a system.

The chakras are like the leaves of a tree: they radiate outward from the same source (the trunk). The power comes from how everything is interconnected and works together as a system. If one of your chakras is out of balance, then it will affect everything else in your life.

There are seven main chakras in the human body that all have their specific purposes and energies. These chakras are located on the back, from base to head. They're also associated with the human body's major organs, and each one of them has a specific color:

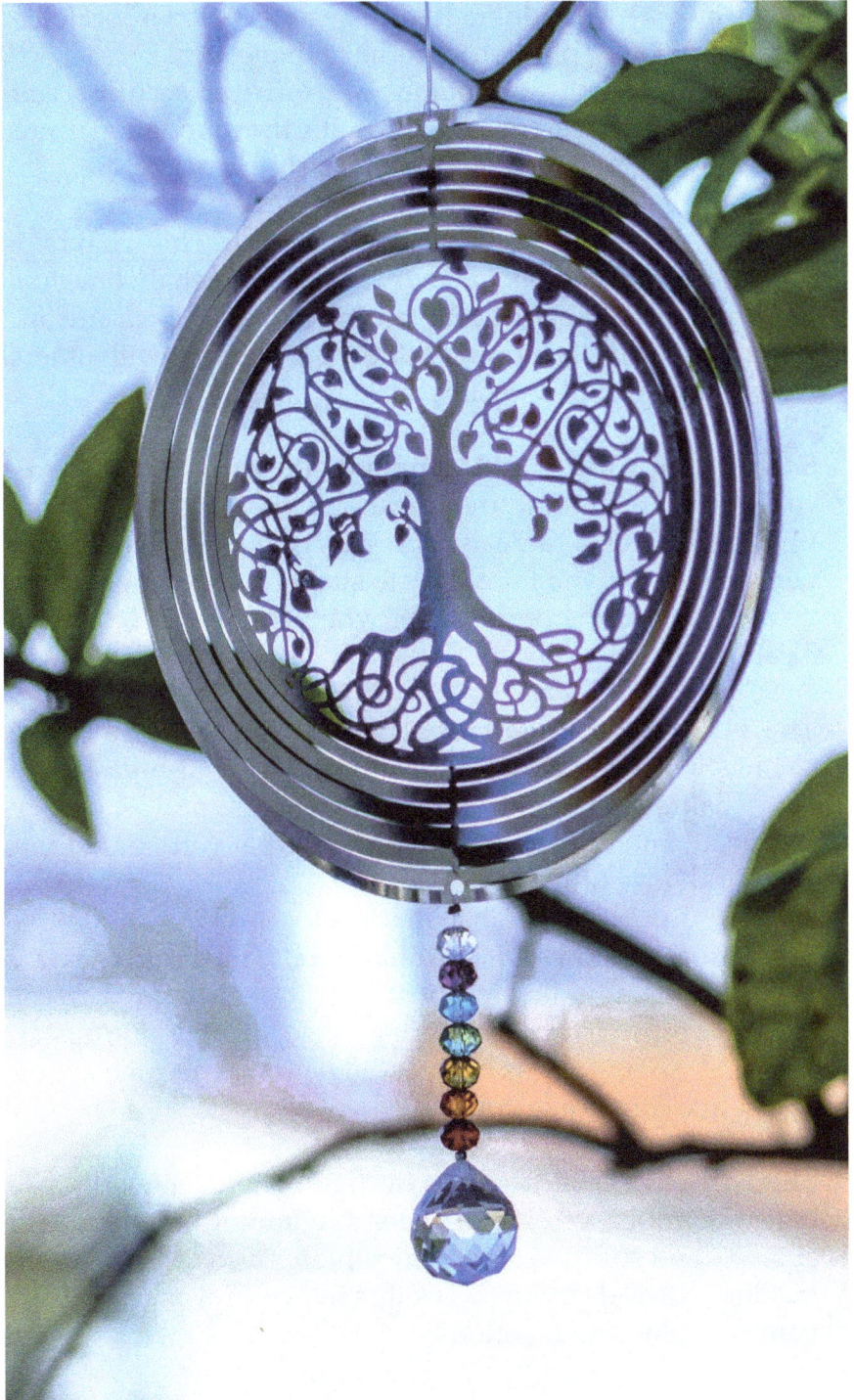

1. **Root Chakra – Muladhara (red):** The root chakra is located at the base of your spine, around the tailbone area. This chakra deals with feelings of intimacy, sex drive, security, self-esteem, and safety in relationships. It's the foundation center of the human body, giving stability and confidence.

2. **Sacral Chakra – Swadhisthana (orange):** This chakra is placed near the tailbone in your lower abdomen (below your belly button). The sacral chakra controls sexual pleasure and creativity as well as forming healthy connections with others. It also helps you find joy in everyday life.

3. **Solar Plexus Chakra – Manipura (yellow):** The solar plexus chakra can be found in the upper abdomen, just below your rib cage. This chakra deals with self-confidence, self-esteem, personal power, and the ability to stand up for oneself. It also helps you find the center when you're confused or feel off balance.

4. **The Heart Chakra – Anahata (green):** The heart chakra belongs in the center of your chest behind your breast bone. This chakra deals with love and compassion, as well as emotional intelligence. It also controls what you put out into the world: love or hate.

5. **The Throat Chakra – Vishuddha (blue):** The throat chakra is located in the middle of your throat. It deals with how you express yourself, from body language to how you speak. Learning to control this chakra will help you become a more expressive communicator.

6. **The Third Eye Chakra – Ajna (indigo):** This chakra is located between your eyes, and it deals with intuition, psychic abilities, and spiritual enlightenment. It's also responsible for making critical decisions, as well as self-control and balancing your thoughts and emotions.

7. **The Crown Chakra – Sahasrara (violet):** The crown chakra is placed near the top of your head. This chakra deals with spirituality, self-love, and letting go of the ego. It allows you to be connected to the cosmos and feel at peace within yourself.

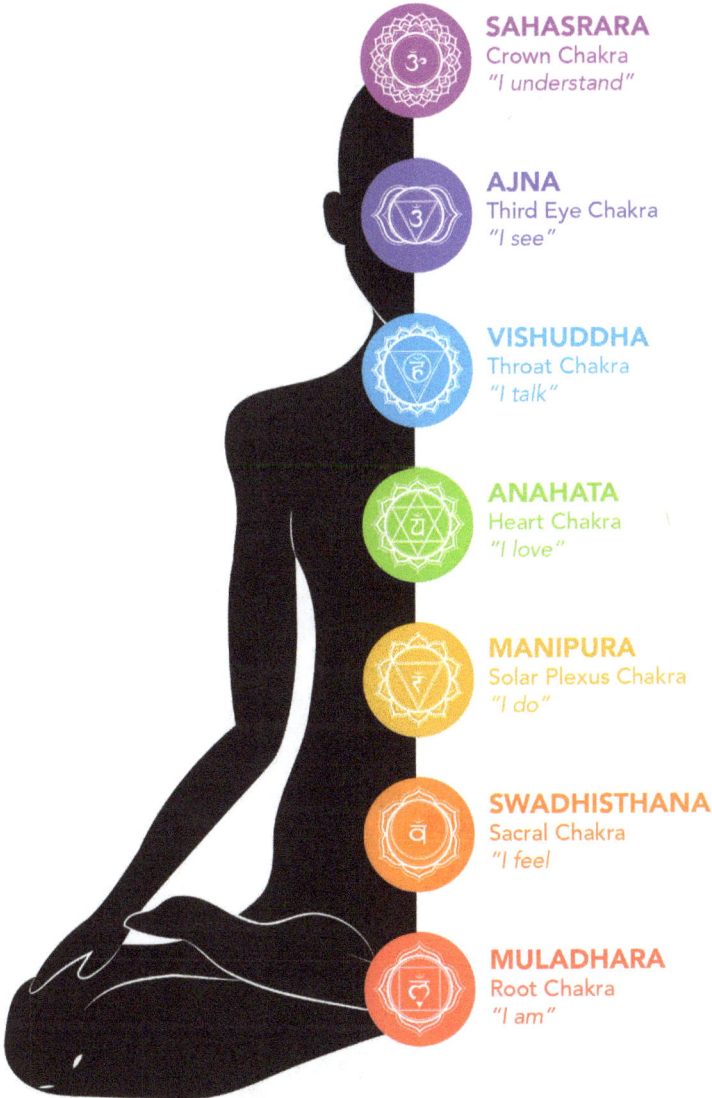

SAHASRARA
Crown Chakra
"I understand"

AJNA
Third Eye Chakra
"I see"

VISHUDDHA
Throat Chakra
"I talk"

ANAHATA
Heart Chakra
"I love"

MANIPURA
Solar Plexus Chakra
"I do"

SWADHISTHANA
Sacral Chakra
"I feel

MULADHARA
Root Chakra
"I am"

~ CHAPTER 3 ~

Complete Yourself With Your partner

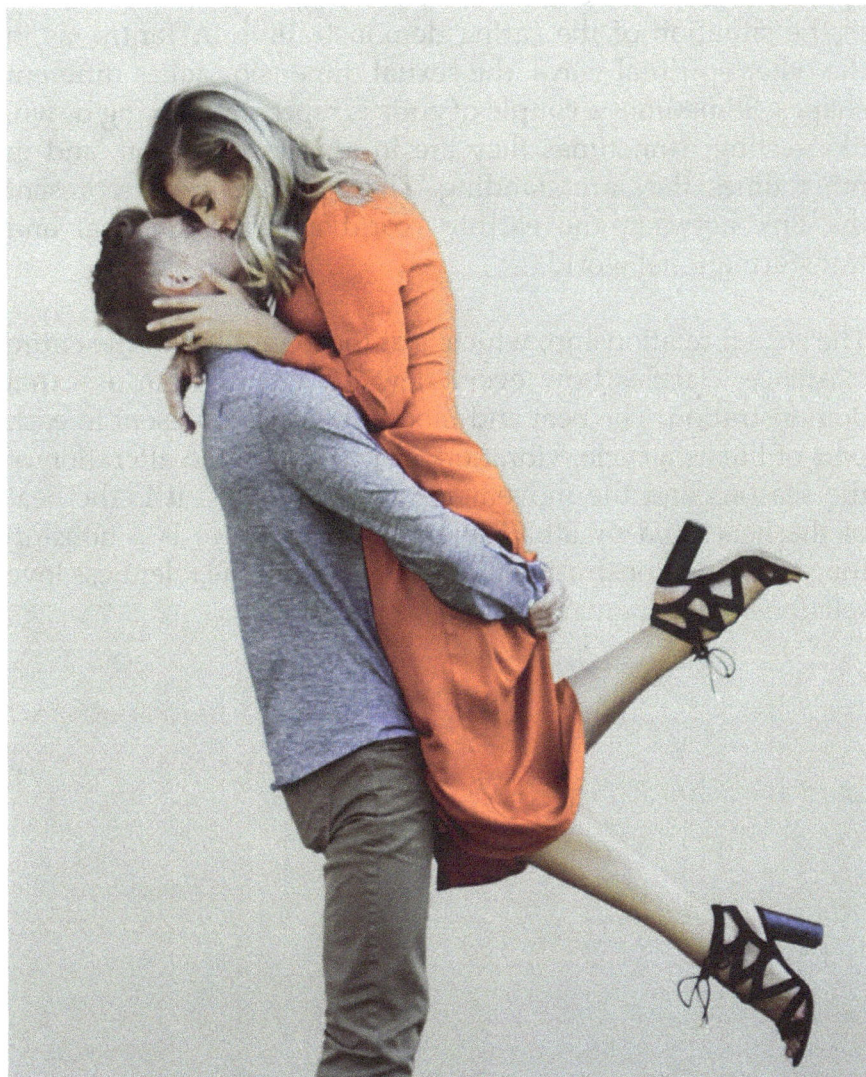

3.1 SEX AS SACRED ENERGY

In numerous, western and eastern cultures, sex is considered one of the most potent sacred energies, second to none. The thought that bound together these ancient cultures was that everything in the universe comes from sexual energy.

In India, Tibet, and China, this assembled vision arrives at its apogee: the divinities are addressed together and frequently in the situation of the caring demonstration. In Tantra, as in the other spiritual ways, the sexual dimension takes different shapes. Sometimes a couple of gods is represented lying down, like resting, sometimes they are in a sitting position, and in other times they are standing. These sacred icons represent the link between the earthly world and the spiritual and transformational world.

The sexual relationship, which is at the beginning of the entire existence, clarifies how every new life comes from a sexual demonstration. The beat and mood of love are present in each part of life as a cycle, vibration, or pulse. It is the alteration of the seasons and the movements of the planets; it is the beat of the heart and breath. Therefore, all presence is a nonstop innovative demonstration that emerges from the relentless love relationship of cognizance and energy.

3.2 Shiva and Shakti

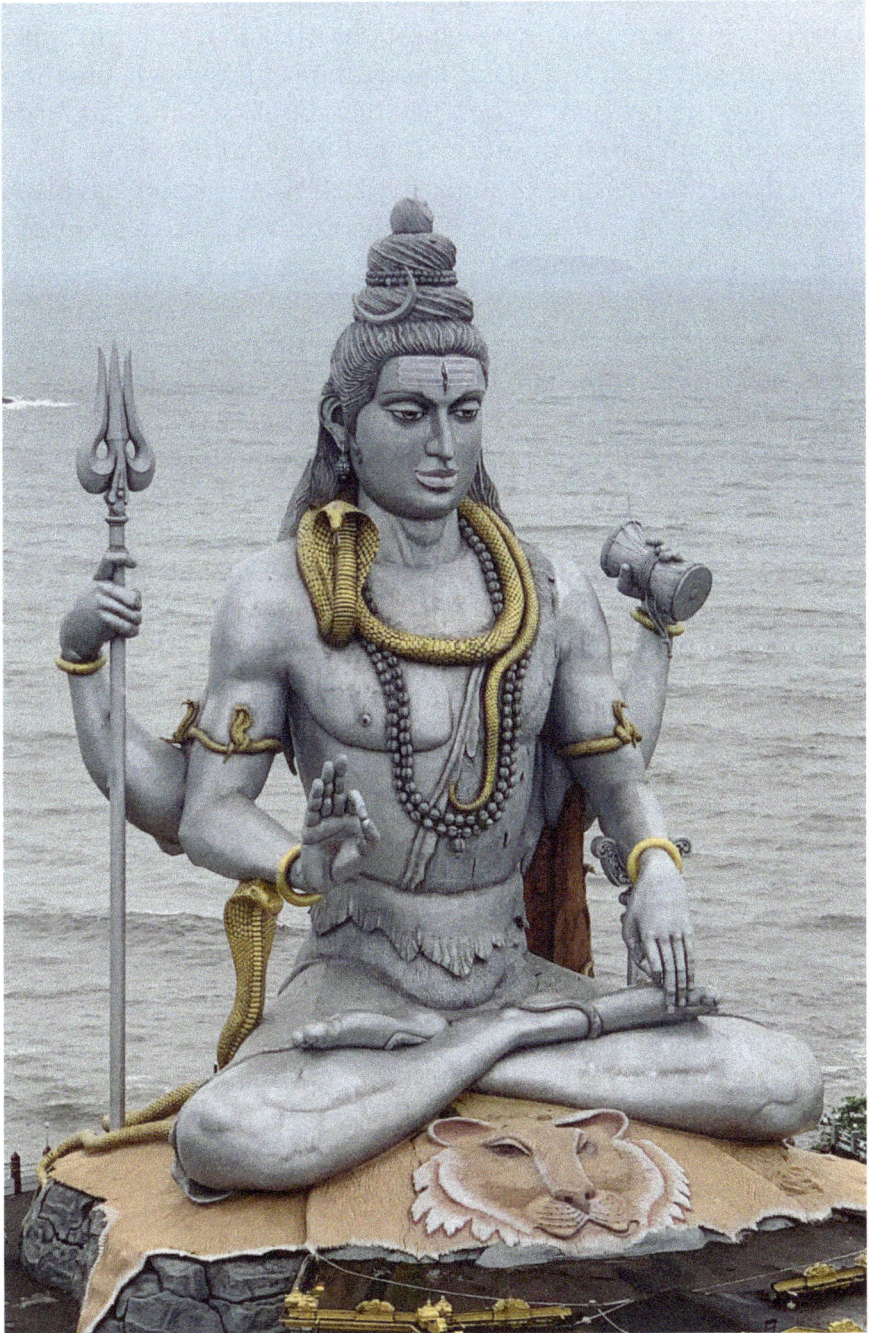

Every culture and religion has its own creation story; most of the ones that I'm familiar with usually narrate an event that occurred at the very beginning of time. This is when creation happens, and everything else happens after that point in time. The Tantra creation story is different; in fact, it refers to creation as an ongoing process. When we talk about creation in tantric philosophy, the first question is not how things have been created but who created them. In Tantra, everything revolves around *Brahman*, the supreme consciousness, and the concept that we are not the subject of our life; Brahman is.

The supreme consciousness is dreaming our existence the entire time and doing with us whatever it desires to do. Brahman is not just the God of the universe, but it is also every particle in it. Tantric religion thinks that all the entities in the universe are all expressions of Brahma. Also, according to Tantra, Brahman is made of two fundamental principles, *Shiva* and *Shakti*. Shiva is also called *Purusa* (consciousness), while Shakti can be called *Prakrti* (energy). Philosophically doesn't mean that God can be broken into two parts. It just means that there are two sides of the same God. We can say that Purusa is the cognitive principle of Brahman while Prakrti is the operative principle of Brahman.

Trying to explain this in just a few words is not simple, but I will give it a try. According to Tantra, God is always observing everything, but at the same time, God is being everything and is doing everything. When God is watching, then Brahman is in the role of Shiva (Purusa), and when is he is doing something, then he is in the role of Shakti (Prakrti). We can see Purusa as something that is static and never changes, while Prakrti is in constant change, and it multiplies. Prakrti acts as a bind for Purusa; It puts Purusa in certain constraints according to Purusa's will. We can say that Shakti (Prakrti) allows Shiva (Purusa) to express itself according to the three Gunas (binding principles): Sattvaguna, Rajoguna, and Tamoguna.

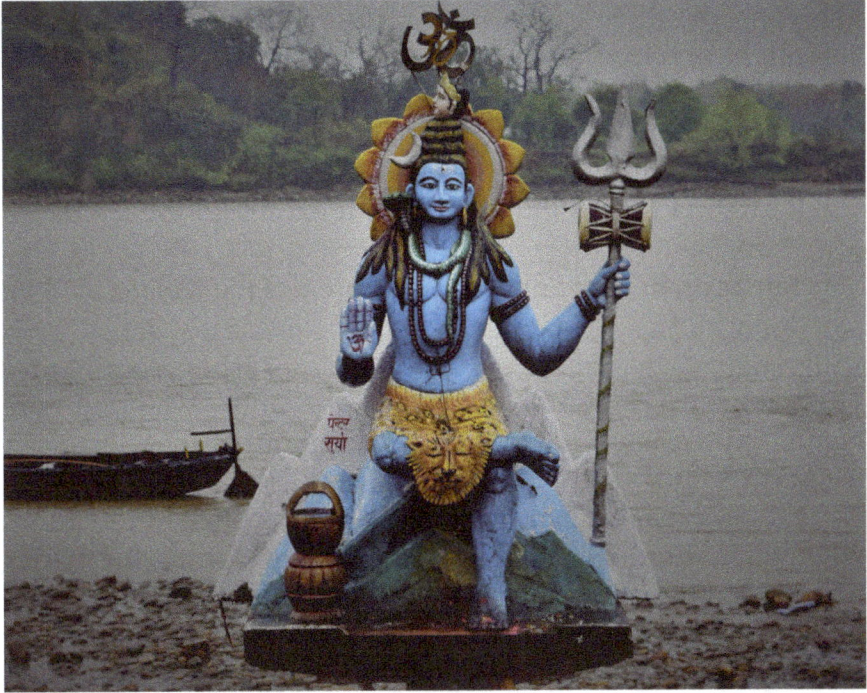

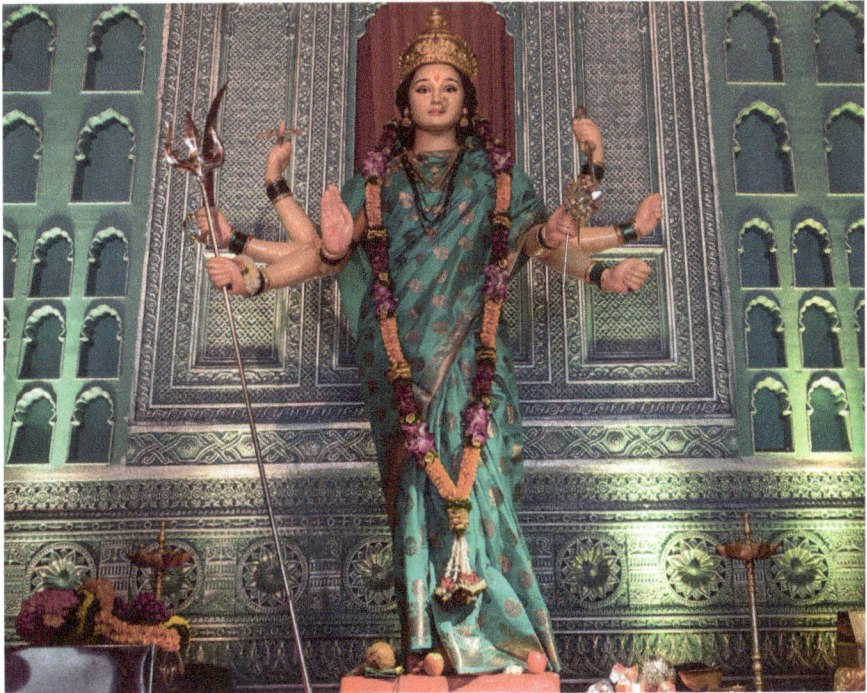

These are the three expressions of Brahman and the qualities you might find in every aspect of the universe.

- **Sattvaguna** means sentient, and it expresses the feeling of "I exist." This is how Shiva becomes aware of itself.
- **Rajoguna** means mutative, and it expresses the feeling of "I do."
- **Tamagun** means static, and it expresses the feeling of "I've done."

These three expressions, "I exist," "I do," and "I've done," are mental expressions, and we can infer that out of consciousness, it comes "mind."

So, if consciousness came first and it lately obtained the mind, what will naturally come next? According to Tantra, the matter was created next. Everything we can see, everything that is part of the universe, was made after consciousness acquired mind.

We can draw a parallel here with the big bang theory. According to this theory, the universe was generated from a single location and is, since then, in constant expansion. According to the Tantra, consciousness is in continuous expansion, obtaining a mind and later turning into the matter.

The big bang theory also says that time and space were the first things to exists before the matter was created, while in Tantra, we say that consciousness and mind came before matter.

These are just some similarities between the big bang theory and tantra, but let's now leave behind the theory of tantric creation to see the relation between Shiva and Shakti in more detail.

According to *Shaivism*, one of the branches of yogic philosophy, we can see Shiva as divine masculine energy while Shakti is considered divine feminine energy. Since Shiva and Shakti are an integral part of Brahman, they are also alive in every man and woman. We can say that everyone has divine masculine traits (Shiva) and divine feminine traits (Shakti); accessing them is not easy, but it can be an enlightening and surprising experience. Shiva is forever in union with Shakti, his divinely feminine consort; the nature of Shiva's energy is steadfast, stable, peaceful, strong, and totally unmoved with complete presence. It represents the state of being unaffected by pain or suffering brought on by the external world.

All the things of creation are generated through the feminine aspect of Shakti; her energy is dance, movement, power, energy, and the freedom to change. We can say that Shiva is a pure being in its stillness while Shakti is pure becoming in all her flow and creativity and her endless opening to possibility. Shakti is fluid, flowing, and powerfully flexible; her energy can be wildly sensual, raw, and expressive.

One of the main differences between their energies is that Shiva's energy is formless, while Shakti's energy can be seen in all things. These two energies are equal and opposite forces; we can't have one without the other, but we will see this concept in more detail in the following chapters.

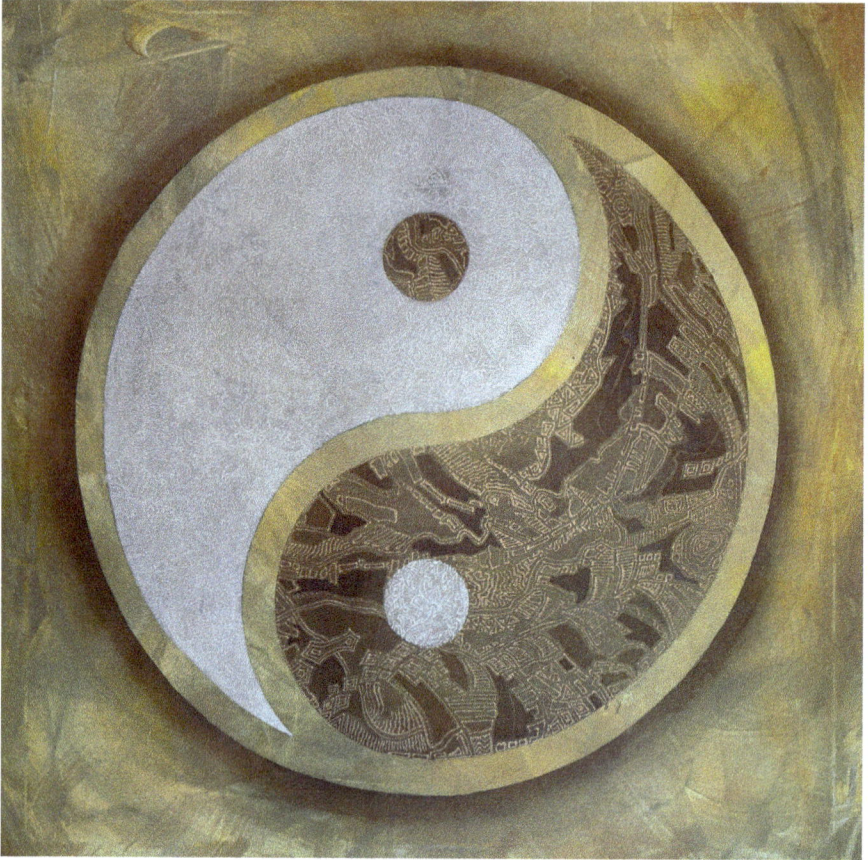

Since the fusion of Shiva and Shakti is the origin of the creation itself, these two entities are sometimes represented together as two halves of the same body, called *Ardhanarishvara*. This image is the synthesis of masculine and feminine energies of everything in the universe. It illustrates how the two forces are inseparable from each other but yet in the perfect balance. This tantric, unitary and transformative vision expanded from India to Tibet and China, where it assumes the image of Tao wherein the two polar powers Yin and Yang in balance. The Taoists' and tantric paths have some similarities: they accept mindfulness as the core of everything. They both recognize the equilibrium of female and male in each element and creature in the universe.

As indicated by the essential tantric standards, sex consolidates female energy and male energy and makes their union a blast, leading the two sides to rise. Reaching the highest pleasure is the final goal. Yet, there are additional halfway objectives, for example, freeing oneself up to love, improving collaboration with the partner, personally feeling the other as though they are one and the other.

To apply what is necessary to allow the couple to open to the Infinite (or possibly part of it), it is fundamental that the two sections are "spellbound," one of Yang (male) energy and the other of Yin (female) energy. The carrier of male energy (Yang) should take on the greatest manly ascribes. His essence is genuine mindfulness and steadiness. The conveyor of female energy (Yin) should remind female ascribes, like imperativeness, attachment to feelings, and disposition to change. Hence, in Tantra, utilization of sensuality is an instrument to rise above. Ladies are attempting to turn out to be more "ladylike" and men more "manly." In Tantra, the male body is full of Yang energy for the most part, and the female body carries Ying energy. They are opposite energies that attract each other, yet, together, they are balancing the universe. The method of the Tao is consistently a path looking for balance, which is possible to achieve only with the harmonization of the outer Yin and yang (the woman and the man) and the inner Yin and yang (in every lover). The outcome acquired is called "Twofold Elevation."

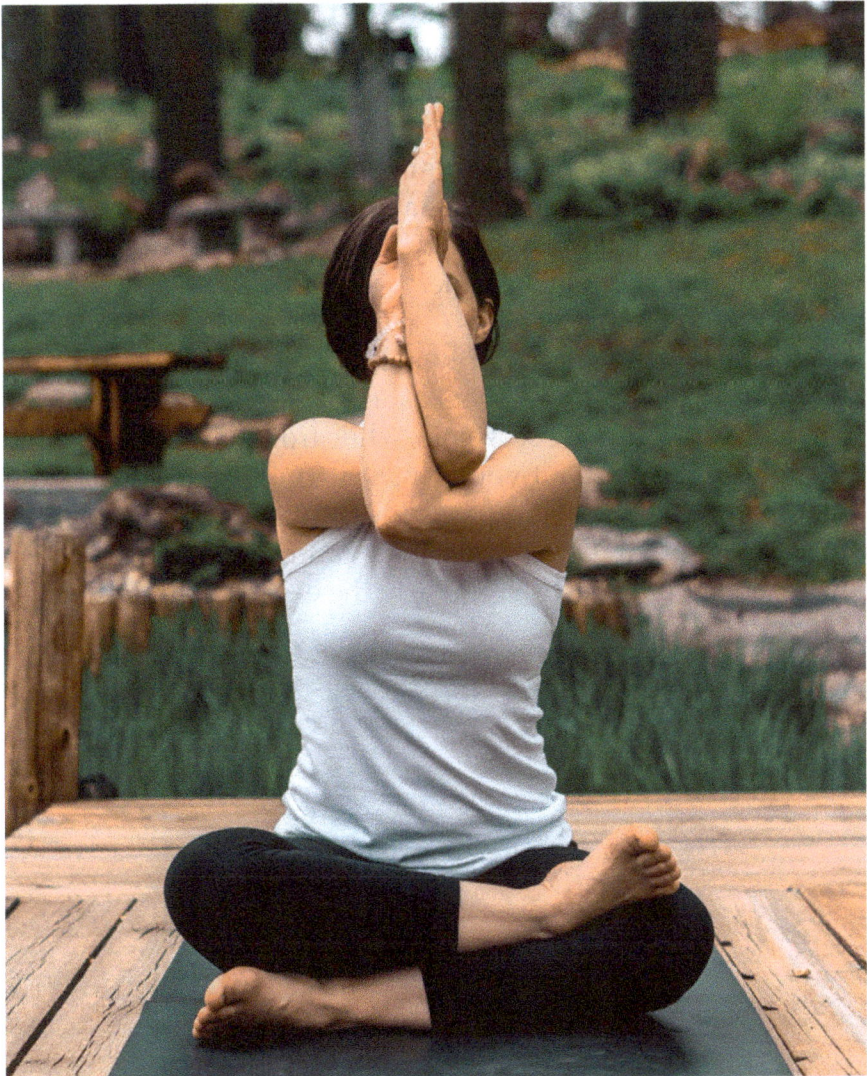

CHAPTER 4

Tantric Yoga

In the past chapters, I introduced the two main branches of tantra: the white tantra and the red tantra (or right and left hand). As already mentioned, the white tantra is a solo path based on yoga and meditation, while the red tantra is based on sexual practices to perform as a couple. They both lead to achieving liberation, but either of them will make you work on different skills and objectives.

The white tantra will help you build more consciousness about yourself and your body, while the red tantra will lead you to create a deeper bond with your partner. While the western neotantra may infer otherwise, the two paths should cooperate to facilitate the final achievement. Chose to walk only one of those paths will make your final goal much more challenging to achieve. Learning Tantric Yoga can make you a better lover, and tantric sex is the opportunity to know more about yourself with the support of your partner.

For this reason, I want to apply in this book some practices for both paths. This chapter will talk about some yoga and breating practices that you exercise in solo, while from the next one, we'll get more in detail about your tantric sexual experience. If you want to get to the hot part sooner, feel free to skip this chapter, but if you are willing to bring your tantric sex to the highest level, you should practice regularly the exercises suggested.

4.1 Tantric Yoga Positions

Yoga is an ancient form of exercise based on *asana* (body postures), meditation, and breathing. This kind of workout will help you build flexibility, strength and it's also an efficient technique for relaxation. Tantric yoga is a form of yoga aligned with Tantra. While tantric and classic yoga share most of their meditation techniques and body position, the main difference is the perception of the body. From a classical yoga perspective, the body is inferior because it belongs to the material world. Instead, in tantric perception, material and spiritual are both parts of the creation and treated at the same level. In conclusion, on a practical level, there is no difference between the two; the only difference is purely theoretical. Therefore, as long as you love your body, you perform tantric yoga when doing this kind of exercise.

The reasons why you should perform yoga in Tantra are both physical and spiritual. First, this kind of exercise helps you build stamina and flexibility that you will need for tantric sex. Last but not least, it will help you set up the correct mindset for Tantra, teaching you how to be relaxed and how to manipulate your breathing for the best living. I selected some exercises that, in my experience, are the most helpful for tantric sex. Of course, you can perform them on your own, but if you are a beginner, my suggestion is to follow a class or find someone to show you the correct posture in performing them. Be aware that doing yoga is a healthy practice, but if you have some particular conditions like pregnancy or circular vascular disease is better that you should ask your doctor's opinion before doing yoga.

1. Cobra pose – Bhujangasama

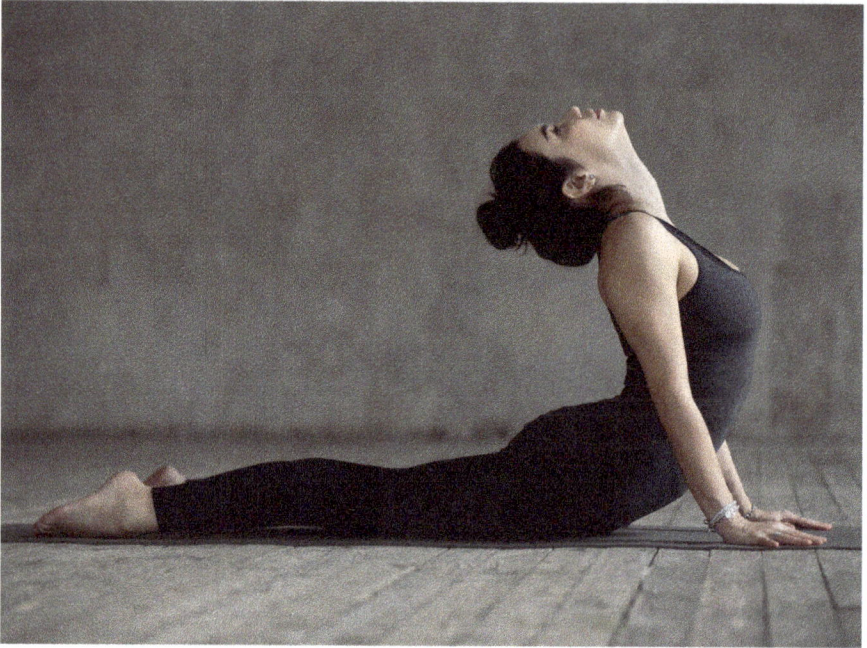

To perform this position, start lying down on your stomach, legs extended, and the toes are pointing straight back and the top of your feet, thighs and pubis firmly into the floor. Spread your hands on the ground under the shoulders and push your torso up. On inhalation, lift your chest off the floor and straighten your arms. Lift the pubis toward the navel and narrow the hips points. When inhaling, your shoulders are moving back, opening your chest. Your shoulders should stay relaxed and the base of your neck soft, while your buttocks are firm but not harden.

Keep this position from 10-30 seconds, breathing easily. After you fully exhale, relaxing your body and going down with your torso. Bend your elbows a little as your chest gets closer to the floor Repeat this sequence from 5 to 10 times. At the end of this practice, you should feel much more light and relaxed!

2. Downward-Facing dog – Adho Mukha Svanasana

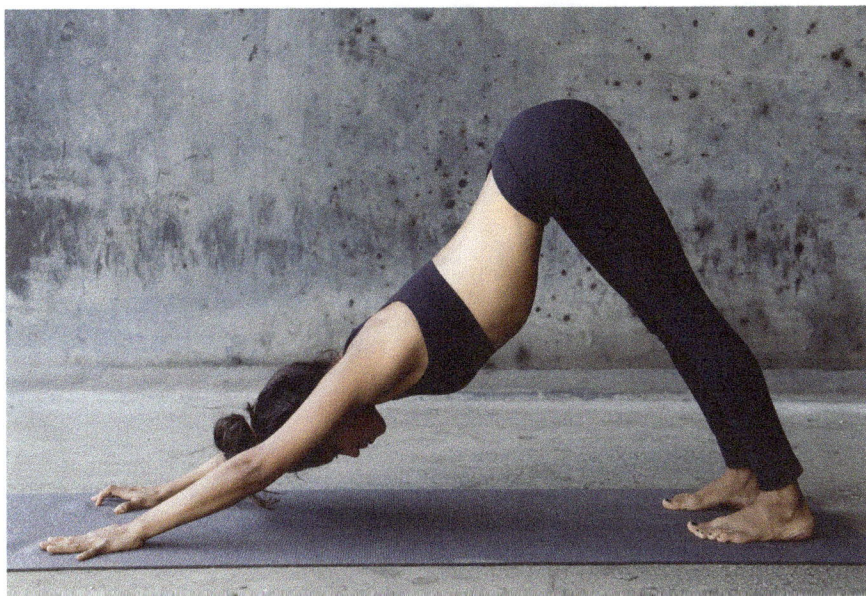

Start this pose in an all-fours position, with the hands slightly forward your shoulders and spread your fingers. Firmly press your hands applying the pressure on the edge of the palms and creating a suction cup in the middle (this status of your hands is called Hasta Bandha). Lift your hips up to bring yourself into an upside-down V pose. In the beginning, keep your knees a bit bent when you adjust your back. Your Shoulders should blade down along the spine, and the base of your neck should stay relaxed. Maintaining your spine stretched, "walk your dog" by alternating bending and straightening your knees.

With each exhalation, root down firmly through your hands; with each subsequent inhalation, send your hips back and up even more. Hold for anywhere from a few breaths to a few minutes, then release. For this position, remember to focus more to keep length in the spine than straight legs, so it's ok to keep your keens a bit bent if you need to feel more comfortable.

3. SUPINE SPINAL TWIST – SUPTA MATSYENDRASAN

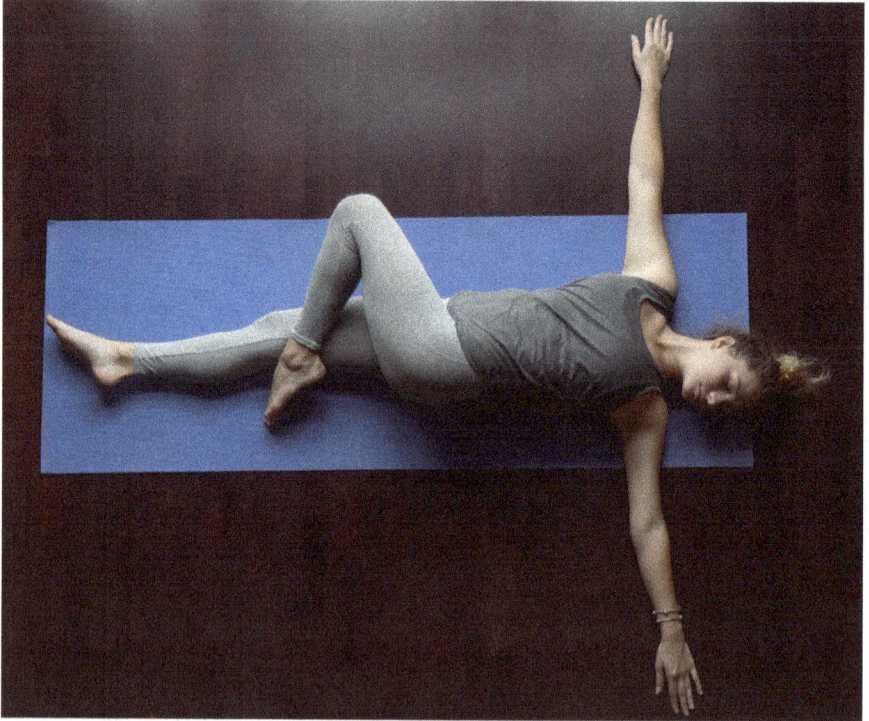

The Supine Spinal Twist stretches the back muscles and realigns and lengthens the spine giving more flexibility and endurance to the subject. Start lying down on your back and bring your arms in a T position, with the palms facing down. Next, bend your right knee over the left side of your body, twisting the spine and low back. Once in this position, use your left hand to push your right knee against the floor; you should feel your thigh and lower back stretching. Your gaze should look in the opposite direction of your knees or toward the ceiling. Keep your shoulders flat to the floor when twisting your body. Keep this position for 6-10 breaths before repeating it with the other side.

4. Warrior 1 – Virabhadrasana I

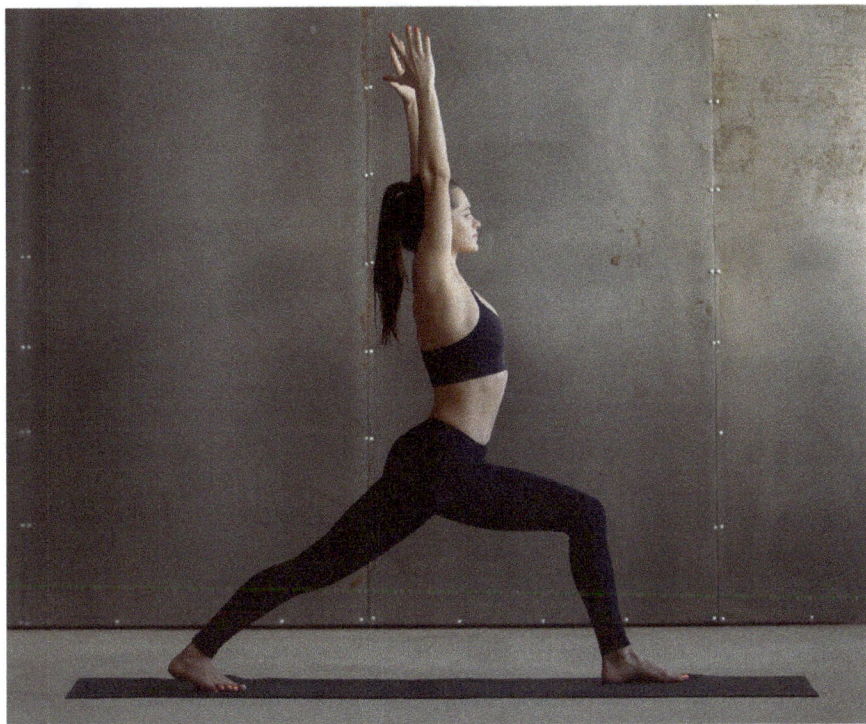

There are three variations for the Warrior Pose, and each of them can be performed to improve your tantric sex. I chose this one because it's ideal for stretching your muscles, and it also helps tone your thighs and butt. It will also improve your stamina and endurance that are always helpful for tantric love.

Start this position standing up straight. Then step your right foot back approximately 45° inward, while your front knee bend at 90° or slightly more. Next, straight your spins and drop your shoulders back while you raise your arms above your head. Your left leg should stay strong as you hold this position for 30 seconds or so. To release, unbend your front knee, centering the torso, and bring your arms down slowly. Repeat the pose bringing back your left leg this time.

5. Plow pose – Halasana

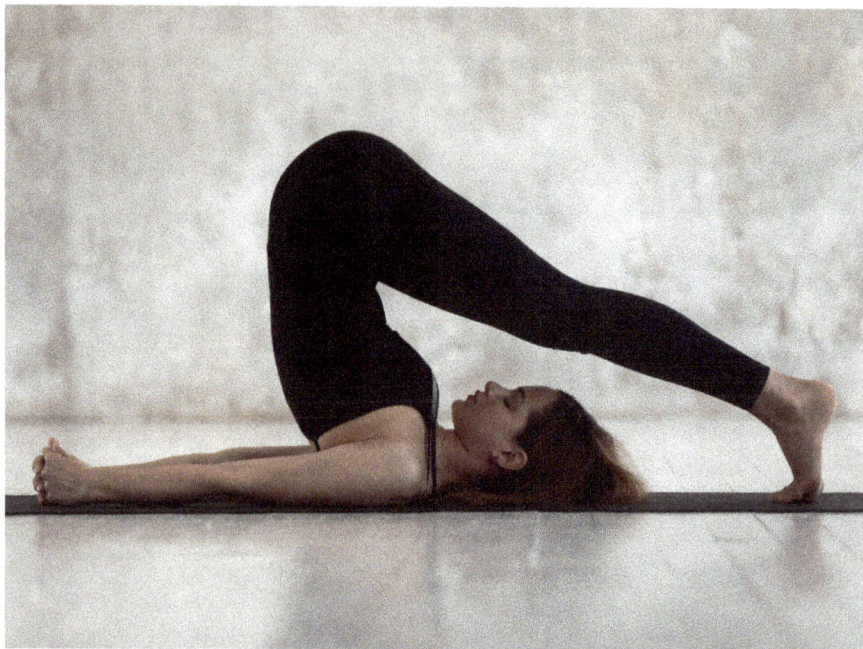

Halasana or Plow (or plough) Pose is an inverted asana that stretches back and shoulders. This pose relaxes the nervous system and relieves stress and fatigue. Consider that this exercise is not a straightforward pose, and you may not get it right at the first attempt. The difficulty level is medium-hight, so it's better if you practice with the previous ones if you are a beginner, and for the first time, it's better if you check with someone that you are in the correct position.

To accomplish this pose, start lying flat on your back with the arms on your sides, hands with palms down, and then extend your legs. When inhaling, use your abdominal muscles to lift your hips and legs. Bring your torso perpendicular to the floor. Keeping your legs extended, slowly lower your toes until touching the floor. If you are struggling to touch the floor, don't worry, you just need some practice; put your toes as lower as you can, keeping the legs extended, and support your back with your hands. If you can reach the floor, then extend your arms and interlace your fingers, pressing your upper arms firmly into the floor. To have this position done correctly:

1. Your Torso is perfectly perpendicular to the floor
2. The legs are extended straight as much as you can
3. There is some space between your chin and the chest and softens your throat. Your eyes should gaze down toward your cheeks.

Once reached the position, hold the pose for up to five minutes. To release, support your backs when returning your legs. Move slowly when rolling down, and if you need, you can bend your knees.

This pose is perfect for letting out your stress, and it's a good exercise for your stamina. It will help you to have better endurance and a relaxed mind.

~ CHAPTER 5 ~
# Breathing

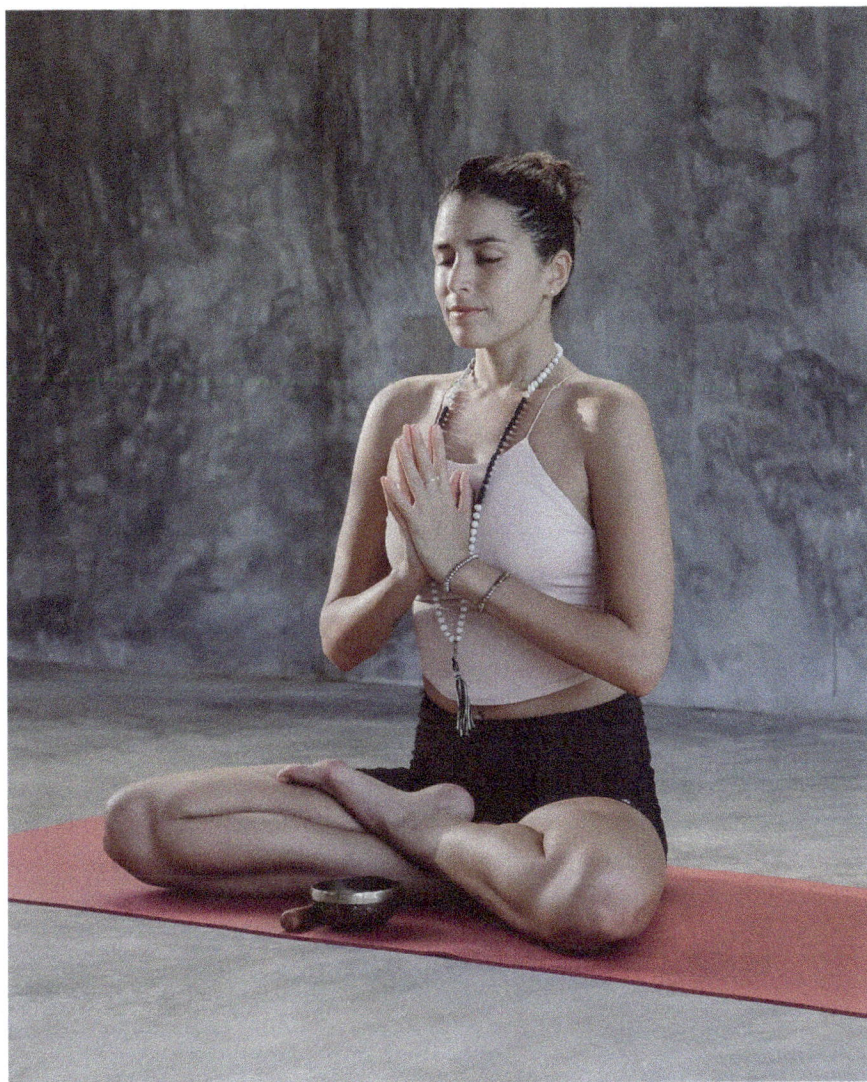

Breathing is an action that comes naturally, and most of the time, people don't even think about it. However, we learn to deal with breath since we get into the world. Without it, we wouldn't be able to stay alive.

Unfortunately, from a very young age, we begin to limit our breath. Remember when your parents screamed at you when you were too loud and too full of energy? We have grown up thinking that being energetic and noisy could cause us trouble, so we soon adjusted our breath to keep it shallow and quiet.

We empower our body with energy through breathing, but this is not necessarily positive; it can also be negative energy. We rarely think about it (or we don't think about it at all), but how we breathe affects our mood and spirit.

You don't have to believe my word; we can do a quick experiment just now. First, try to take a shallow and short breath; don't you feel small and maybe a bit off? Sometimes when I do it, I can perceive a veil of sadness to which I cannot attribute an origin. Now, try again with a deep and long breath. You have to breathe with your chest and not your stomach. Don't you feel much better? More energized and in control?

With breath, we can regulate our mood and recharge our bodies. In Tantra, mastering the breath is the most efficient way to access your chakra and elevate your spirit to illumination.

I suggest using this technique even in everyday life. From now on, try to pay attention to your breathing and if you feel tired and stressed, take a minute to breathe deeply and recharge your body. Your troubles and issues won't change depending on your breathing, but your perspective will.

5.1 TANTRA BREATHING & PRANAYAMA

Pranayama is the practice adopted in yoga that focuses on controlling the breath. *Prana* is the Sanskrit word meaning "life energy" while *yama* means "control"; so, the whole world pranayama means "control of life energy," and sometimes you can see it also translated as "extension of breath." The ancient yogis recognized how breathing was essential for our body to survive. So, they practiced some techniques to regulate breathing, releasing stress, and increasing physical and mental health.

In tantric sex, breath is essential to connect with another person. If you want to synchronize with your partner (and since you are doing tantric sex, you do want), you must match your breaths. Try to inhale and exhale together; you need to do it intensely and remember to use your chest and not your belly. Breath is like the rhythm of life, and if you are connected with breath, you are dancing together.

Breathing is one of the manners in which Tantra varies from different kinds of sex. With tantric breathing, you center around your accomplice's breathing. Once in a while, it's simply staying there and allowing your bodies to move with each other.

When you practice breathing techniques, stay focused on your respiration. In this status, your mind might move to other matters; it is not simple, but you will be able to master your thoughts after some practice. You have to keep thinking that your current center is breathing with your partner, and nothing else has to interfere.

Keep your thoughts far from the orgasm too. At this point, you don't have to stress yourself about the result. If you relax and stay connected with your partner, the rest will come naturally. Enjoy the moment and work on giving a fun, vivid involvement to the individual you're offering yourself.

Breath is the focal core of all Tantra, and breathing is a way to help free the brain, body, and spirit. At the point when you center around your breathing, you'll feel the sensations significantly more intense, and you'll feel more joyful too.

Achieving the perfect synchronization with your partner through breath may sound easy, but it's more complicated than it seems.

Usually, you're on different frequencies, yet the reflective idea of breathing, performed by you and your partner, considers both of you to remain on a similar frequency and thus, build a more profound connection.

5.2 BREATHING TECHNIQUES

Before introducing some pranayama lessons, I want to provide a few breathing exercises that you can perform to improve the connection with your partner.

Calm Breathing

Calm breathing, sometimes called diaphragmatic breathing, is a technique that helps you slow down your breathing when feeling stressed or anxious. This technique allows you to dominate your feelings and overcome anxiety, but it does require some practice to apply it correctly. All breathing techniques require your body to be straight and sitting upright because this posture increases the capacity of your lungs to fill with air. To perform this technique, sit straight, relax your shoulders and take a slow breath through your nose; you must inhale using your diaphragm or abdomen for about 4 seconds. Next, hold your breath for 1 or 2 seconds, then exhale slowly through the mouth for about 4 seconds. Wait a couple of seconds before repeating. If you want to practice with this technique, do about 6-8 breathing cycles every day. Breathing to your nose is a technique used to awake the Ajna Chakra.

Active Cycle of Breathing Technique (ACBT)

This technique is a 3 phase cycle that helps clear mucus from the lungs.

The first phase is **Breathing control**. Like in the previous exercise, sit straight and relax your shoulders. Next, take a gentle breath inhaling through your nose, and exhale slowly through your mouth using the lower part of your chest. To help yourself to improve the execution, you can put one hand on your stomach as you breathe. If it's difficult for you to exhale with an open mouth, you can purse your lips together to create backpressure in the airways that stents the airway open longer. Repeat breathing control for five breaths before moving forward. This phase helps you to relax your airways.

The second phase is the **Chest expansion exercise**. Place your hands onto your ribs cage, then take a long and deep breath in through the nose. Hold your breath for one-two seconds before releasing it with a long gentle breath out through the mouth. During this phase, you should focus on the movements of your ribs that are contracting and expanding during the exercise. Again, you can exhale with an open mount or pursing your lips together to make it easier. Repeat this phase for five breaths.

The last phase is called the **Forced expiration technique**. This phase forces the mucus out of your lungs, so you don't need this phase for relaxation, but you can use it to clear your airways. For this last part, you can mimic steaming a window or a mirror; if you want, you can use your hand in front of you to visualize one of the two. First, take a breath in through the nose, and then open your mouth and huff the air out. You can perform this one in two ways: take a long breath in and a short and quick exhalation, or inhale quickly and breath out slowly. Repeat five times, then complete the cycle with a cough to clear your lungs.

4-7-8 breath

This technique works amazingly to relieve physical and mental pressure. It is suggested to execute this breathing exercise while facing your partner; this will help to synchronize your breaths. Before starting the breathing pattern, adopt a comfortable sitting position and place the tip of the tongue on the tissue right behind the top front teeth. You can do this with your accomplice while holding each other's hand, focusing only on your breathing.

Breathing cycle:
- Breath in for 4 seconds
- Hold your breath for 7 seconds
- Exhale for 8 seconds
- Repeat the cycle four times

5.3 Pranayamas – some effective breathing exercises

Pranayama is a way of reaching higher states of consciousness and is an excellent practice to keep the body and mind healthy. In this section, I selected three of the most effective pranayama techniques. They will help you to calm your mind and to find focus while you are breathing.

When you practice yoga and breathing techniques for the first time, you should do it with the guidance of a knowledgeable teacher. Do not attempt any breathing and yoga exercise if you have a respiratory condition or pregnant without consulting your doctor first. Stop the exercise if you become faint or dizzy. If you have any medical concerns, talk with your doctor before practicing yoga and breathing techniques.

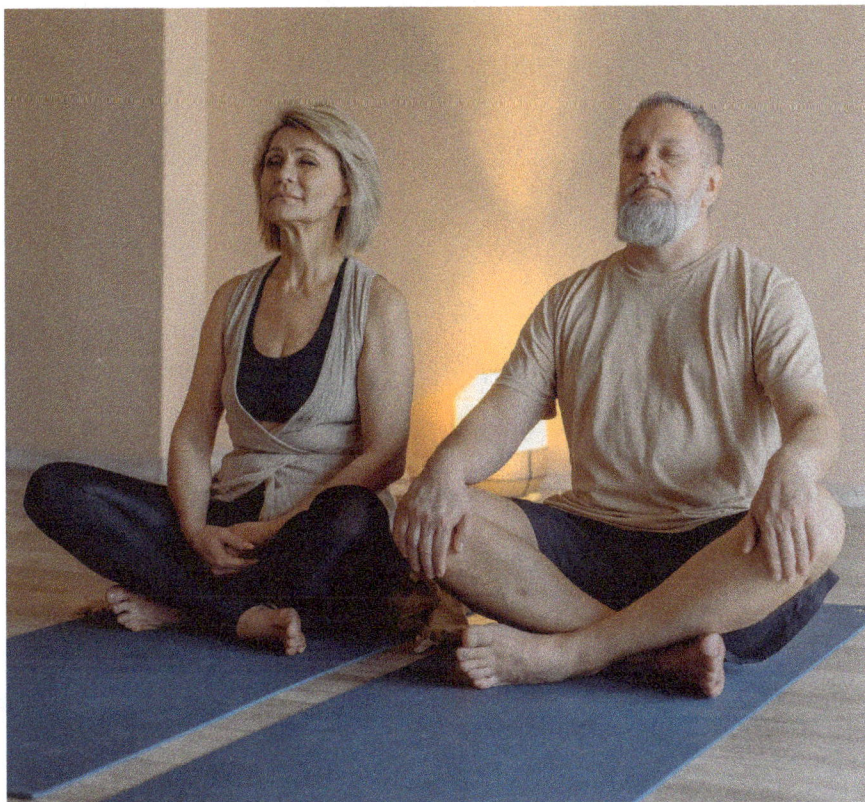

Bhastrika Pranayama – Bellows Breath

Bhastrika, or "bellows breath," is a traditional breathing exercise in yoga that helps to increase *prana* (energy) in your body. This technique helps to remove excess congestion in the lungs and brighten the mind. If you haven't tried this method before, you can stop in the middle and pause from 15 up to 30 seconds. Make sure to listen to your body during the practice. Bellows breathing is a safe practice, but if you feel light-headed in any way, take a pause for a few minutes while breathing naturally. Then, when the discomfort passes, try another round of bellows breathing, slower and less intense.

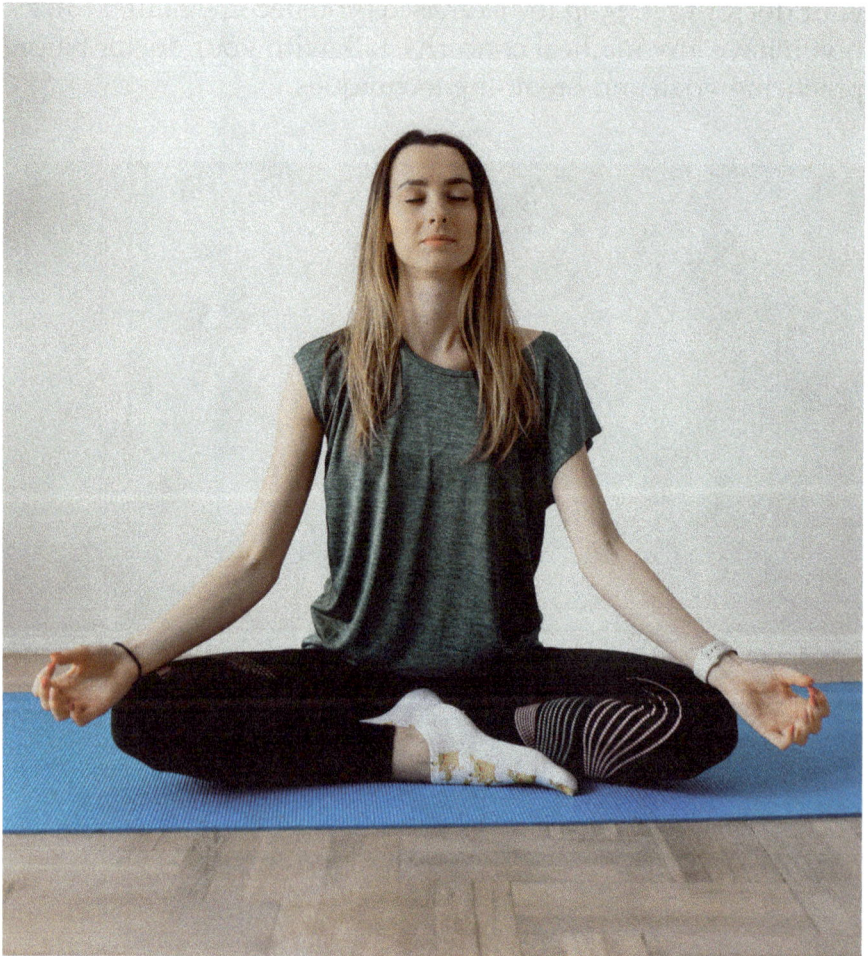

To perform Bhastrika:
- Sit up tall, relax your shoulders.
- Take a few deep breaths in and out from your nose.
- With each inhale, expand your belly fully as you breathe.
- As you breathe out, feel the pelvic floor lifting, which helps bring blood flow to that region.
- Keep your head, neck, shoulders, and chest still while your belly moves in and out.
- After 27 rounds of Bhastrika, take a full breath in and hold, retaining the breath.
- With your hands, clamp the abdominal muscles at the lower abdomen and, as you keep the breath, lift and lower the head gently 3-5 times.
- Release the clamp and breath normally.

You can attempt this technique with your partner facing each other and try to copy each other's moves, but if one of you is in discomfort, try to slow it down.

Nadi Shodhana and Anulom Vilom Pranayama

Known as *Alternate nostril breathing*, it's a technique used for relaxation. This technique involves holding one nostril closed with your thumbs while inhaling. Then, keeping the other nostril closed while exhaling. This practice is ideal for balancing the breath, and if done regularly, it can improve circulation and calm the nervous system.

To perform *Anulom Vilom*:
- Sit in Padmasan (sitting with your legs crossed but both your feet are on your thighs) or if you feel more comfortable, sit with your legs crossed. Rest your hands and your knees and relax your shoulders.
- Close the right nostril with the right thumb while inhaling from the left one.
- Breath in expanding your lungs as much as possible.
- When switching from inhalation to exhalation, remove

the thumb from your right nostril and use your middle finger to close your left nostril. Then exhale, releasing all the air in your lungs.

- Repeat this process for five minutes keeping your focus on your breath.

Once you get used to the *Anulom Vilom*, you can proceed with the next level, which is called *Nadhi Sodhana*. This technique is very similar to the previous one but with two differences. This time, you inhale through the left nostril and breath out through the right. Additionally (and most important), you need to hold your breath for a minute or so between your inhalation and exhalation. Repeat this cycle for 3 or 5 minutes.

As the Anulom Vilom, the Nadhi Sodhana helps relax your mind and body, and it's an ideal exercise for a healthy heart.

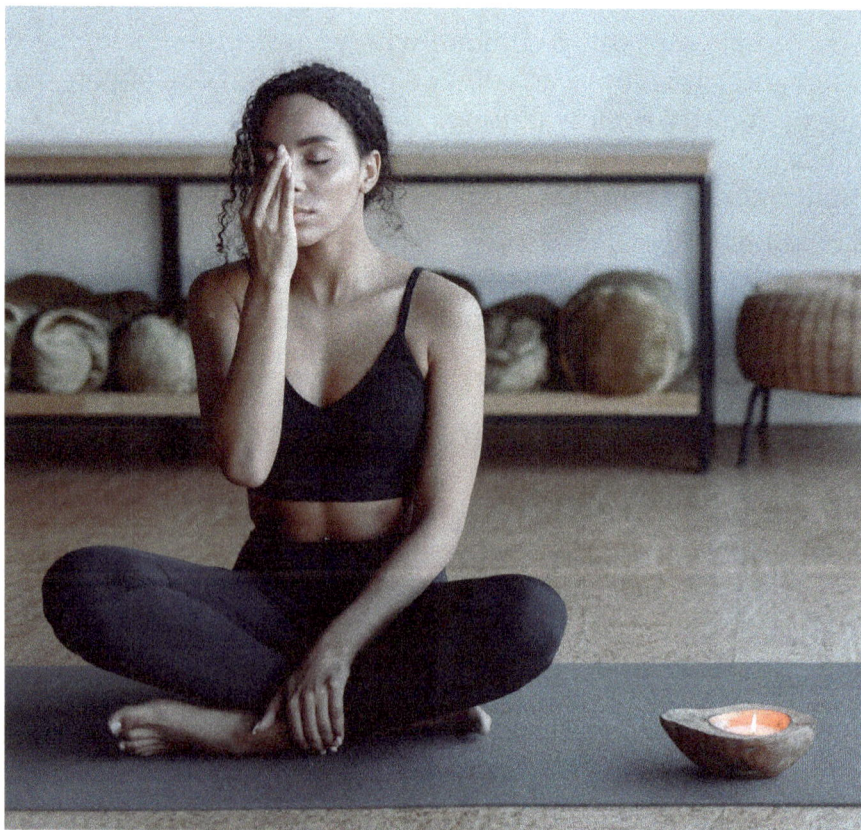

Ujjayi Pranayama

Ujjayi Pranayama is one technique that helps to relax your brain and warm the body. The Sanskrit word ujjayi means "conquer," "being victorious," but because of the sound created when performed correctly, it is also referred to as "ocean breath." Ujjayi encourages the full expansion of the lungs while slightly contracting your throat and breathe through your nose. When practicing Ujjayi Pranayama, be careful not to tighten your throat.

To perform Ujjayi Pranayama:

- Sit in the Easy Pose (or Sukhasana pose - sitting on the floor crossing your legs and having your back straight). Relax your shoulders and close your eyes.
- Let your mouth drop open slightly. Inhale and exhale deeply through your mouth. When exhaling, softly whisper the sound "ahhh" while slightly contracting the back of your throat.
- When you got comfortable with your exhalation, try to maintain the constriction of the throat even when you breathe in. You should notice an "ocean waves" sound coming from your breath if you do this properly.
- When you get comfortable with this breathing and position, you can try to close your mouth and breathe only through your nose. Keep the constriction in your throat like you were doing when the mouth was open. The "ocean sound" should keep coming from your breath. When you get comfortable breathing through your nose, direct the air over your vocal cords, across the back of your throat.
- Concentrate on the sound of your breath; it should be soft and gentle. When breathing in, fill your lungs to their fullest expansion and empty them when you exhale.

Start practicing Ujjayi for five minutes per day; for more profound meditation, increase your time to 15 minutes. Once you get familiar with this breathing technique; also, you can apply Ujjayi while doing yoga.

~ CHAPTER 6 ~
# Preparation

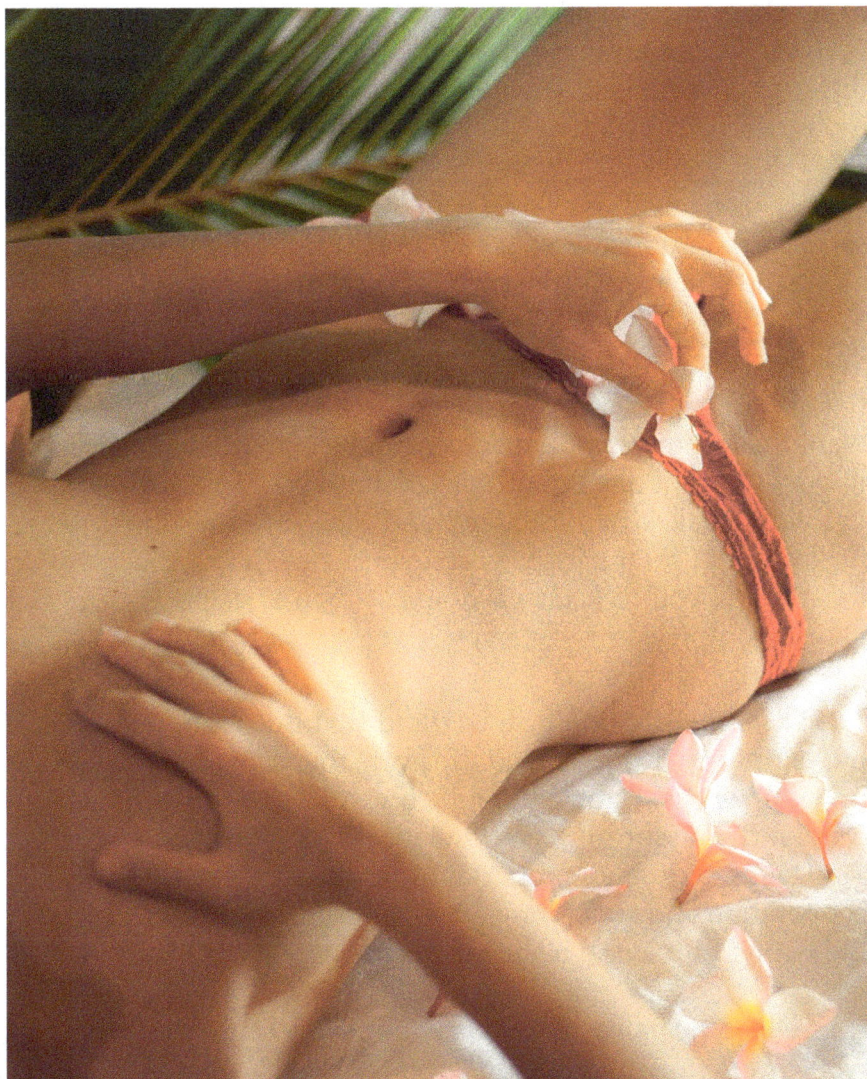

So far, we came across the theoretical part of Tantra, exploring its meaning and its history. But the best part has yet to come because, finally, we are going to learn some practical techniques. It should be clear until now how important is sex in Tantra, but before mastering the "act of love," you need to learn some tactics that will help you and your partner get the most delightful experience.

First, it is essential to focus on your body and the development of sexual activity to advance energy flow.
Secondly, communication during love can't be denied or interrupted. In tantric sex, one shouldn't hesitate to communicate their pleasure at 100%.

At long last, breath is also an excellent alliance to accomplishing satisfaction. You can use some breathing exercises to perform along the whole circle of sexual affectivity for better outcomes.

Talk with your partner
Before starting, ensure that you and your accomplice both want to attempt this. Tantric sex can be a great experience, but it won't work if one or both of you have some hesitation. Keep in mind, it takes two to tango, and that goes for tantric sex as well. Going for tantric sex is an experience that you have to do together. If you're keen on doing it, you need to ensure that your accomplice is in the same spot as you are.

The vast majority don't understand that this is something that the partner may not be ready for yet. You may think beginning immediately is a good thought but forcing your partner will only add pressure on your relationship. Tantra is a process that takes time and preparation, so don't rush it. You need cooperation and synchronization for doing it, and starting with the wrong foot won't be beneficial.

If you're rehearsing tantric sex, yet your partner is not, you won't be able to coordinate because the two of you would move to a different rhythm. If you don't synchronize, one will encounter orgasm early and try to slow down, while the other will rush to catch up. With this dysfunctionality, you won't be able to be one and the other, like Shiva and Shakti, so you'll never reach the greatest pleasure.

Anyway, it shouldn't be challenging to convince your partner. Tantra is an experience that brings to the couple more intimacy and energy. Whatever is the status of your relationship, Tantra is the better way to spice it up. So, all considered, if you open your mind to this path, it will take you to places where you have never been before.

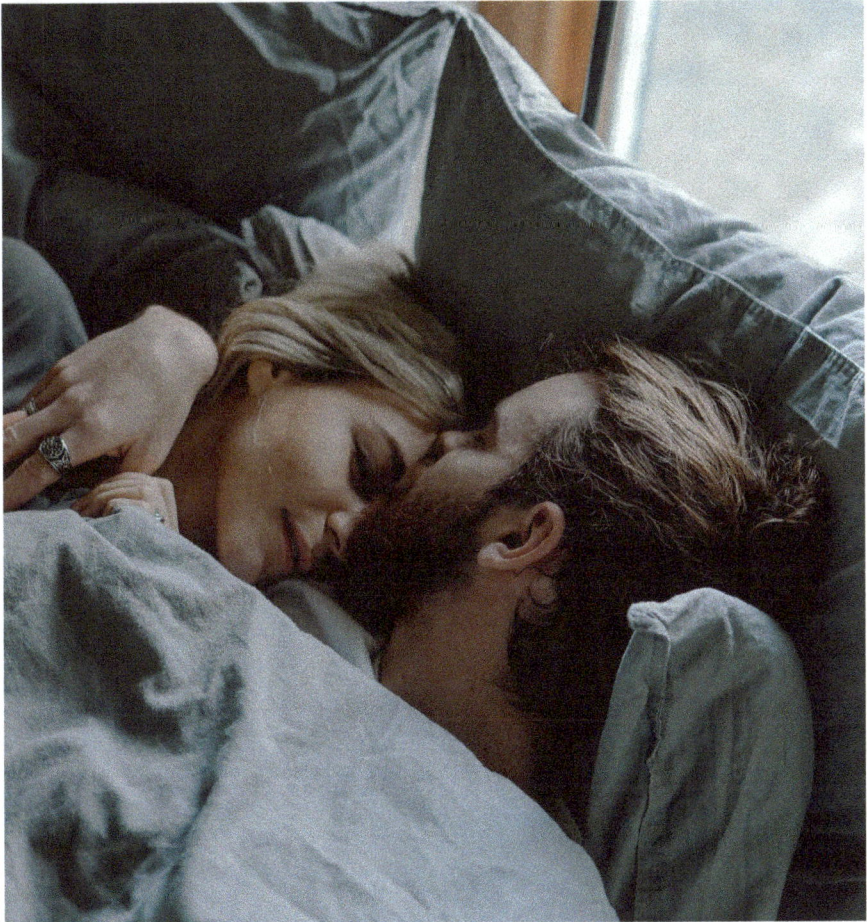

Prepare your body

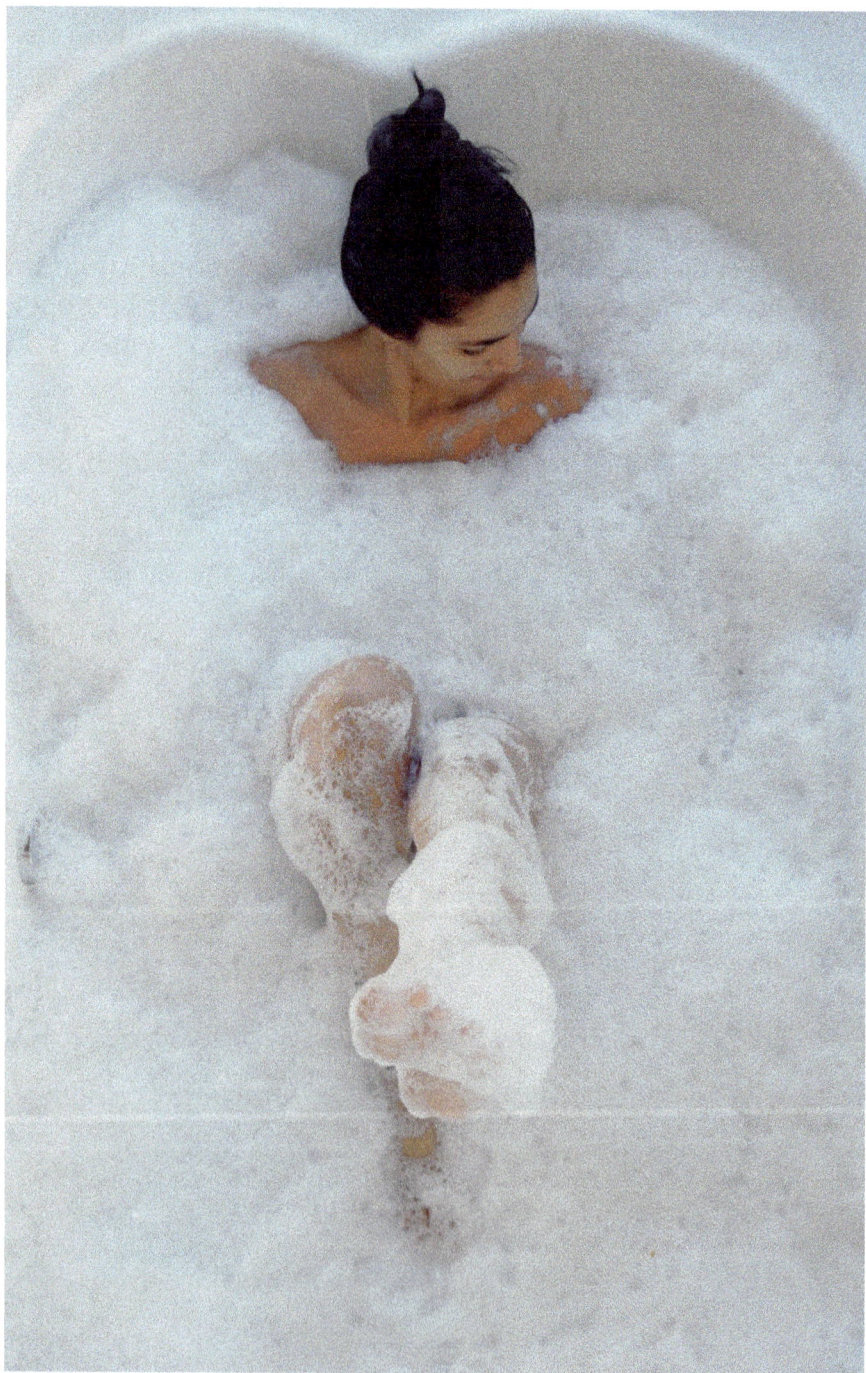

Preparing your body for the Tantra experience is an excellent practice because it will help you relax and recharge your energy. It can also be a grand affair if you and your partner decide to do it together.

There are several options to prepare your body: doing yoga or meditation, practice your breath, showering, and massaging your body. These alternatives have the purpose of taking you to relaxation and losing the tension accumulated during the day. You don't have to do them all; pick up what fits you most.

Although yoga, meditation, and breathing exercise should be considered hobbies rather than actions to apply just before lovemaking. You can use them before sex if they make you feel regenerated, but I recommend doing something that can make you feel good and recharged.

What I like to do most for my preparation is having a long bath. The warm water and the scents help me recharge my spirit, and when I do it with my partner, I feel more connected with him because I am sharing one of the experiences that I like most.

Preparing the body with your partner is not only a great way to build more intimacy, but you can use this situation to do things that would be difficult to do alone. For instance, you can ask your partner to make you a massage, so you don't have to stress out for doing this yourself, and you can fully enjoy the relaxation.

When you get ready together, I suggest taking turns. Allow your partner to help you to relax, let them do a massage, or ask them to refresh your back, and when they have fished, it's your turn to return the favor. During each turn, don't be afraid to give the feedback that you need to. It's ok to tell your partner what they should do better, which will help them give you what you want.

Communication

Agreeing to initiate the tantra path together is not the only step in communication. It may sound redundant in the relationship, but this aspect is a valuable key for tantric sex.

If you want to achieve the highest orgasm, you need to let your partner know what you like so that they can give you the best pleasure. In the same way, you need to listen to the other attendant's lead to provide them the highest gratification.

Don't wait until the end of the session to explain your needs. You have to keep the communication going at every stage of the sexual encounter.

Prepare the atmosphere

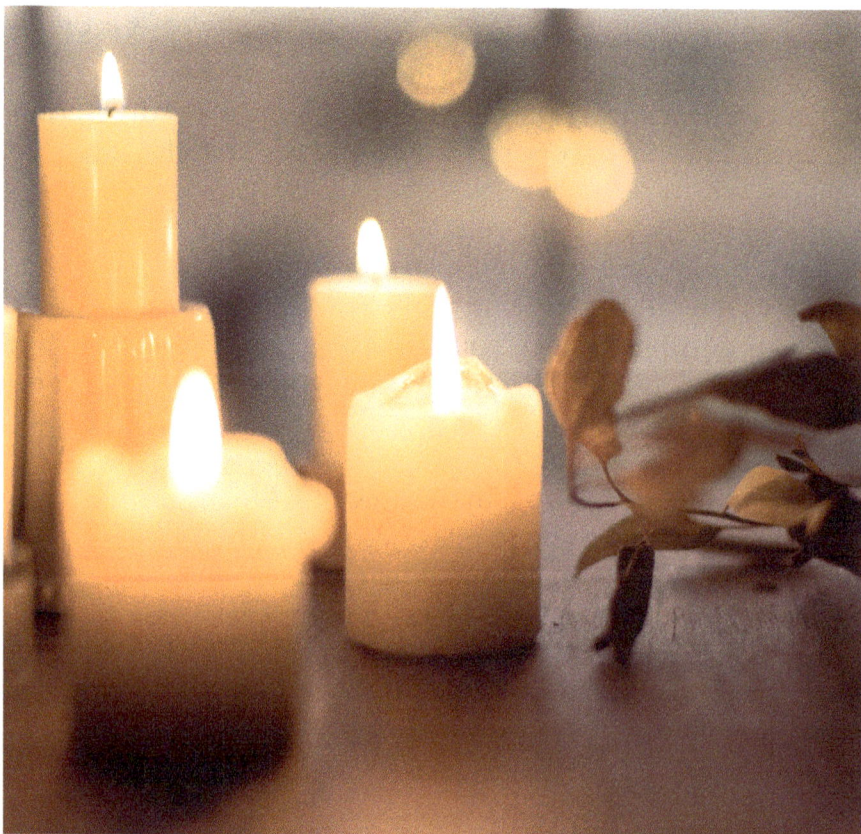

Even if this may sound secondarily important, setting the room where you will share the act of love is a great tip to make you feel more confident and get in the right mood.

Make sure that the room has everything you need to make yourself and your partner comfortable. Prepare the bed, or use a soft carpet if you prefer. Check that you have enough pillows, you don't necessarily have to use them, but it's good to have them around if you feel you need them. They are also helpful allies in case you want to adjust your position if you feel uncomfortable.

Feel free to add candles, flowers, and petals if you think they will help to set the atmosphere, but make sure that they won't be in the way during the performance. Another essential element is light. I don't recommend having tantric sex in the darkness because it will negatively affect your senses and impact your ability to synchronize with your partner.

For tantric sex, the best illumination is a soft light. You can use the lamps for the bedsides or, even better, turning some candles on. If you decide to use the candles, don't use too many of them, a couple would be enough, and please, be careful to put them in a safe place.

Possibly, avoid the colored light, especially the red one. It may look sensual, but red is the most inadequate color for relaxation. This suggested type of illumination, aside from being more romantic, helps concentrate on what is in front of us without disrupting the flow of energies.

The scent is also a valuable component in your room. Most people usually underestimate the power of smell, but it's a valid stimulator for love and relaxation. Scented candles may help to cover this point too, or you can make use of incense. If you are missing both, using some perfume to lightly scent the linens will do just fine.

Diet

In general, a healthy diet is suitable for longer life. This component is also suggested for Tantra because it will help you stay in the right shape to achieve advanced sexual positions. Sure, you don't have to follow a specific diet if you don't want to. And I also don't recommend trying any advanced position before you and your partner have built enough experience to move to a higher step. Anyway, my suggestion is to have a light meal when you are approaching the tantra event. Also, make sure to give your body enough time to digest and enough calories to support the performance. In some ways, it is good to approach the tantric relationship as a sport and provide our bodies with the most suitable nutrients.

Personally, I prefer to have a light meal made of white meats and vegetables and bring some peeled fruit to the room in the case of a long and tiring session.

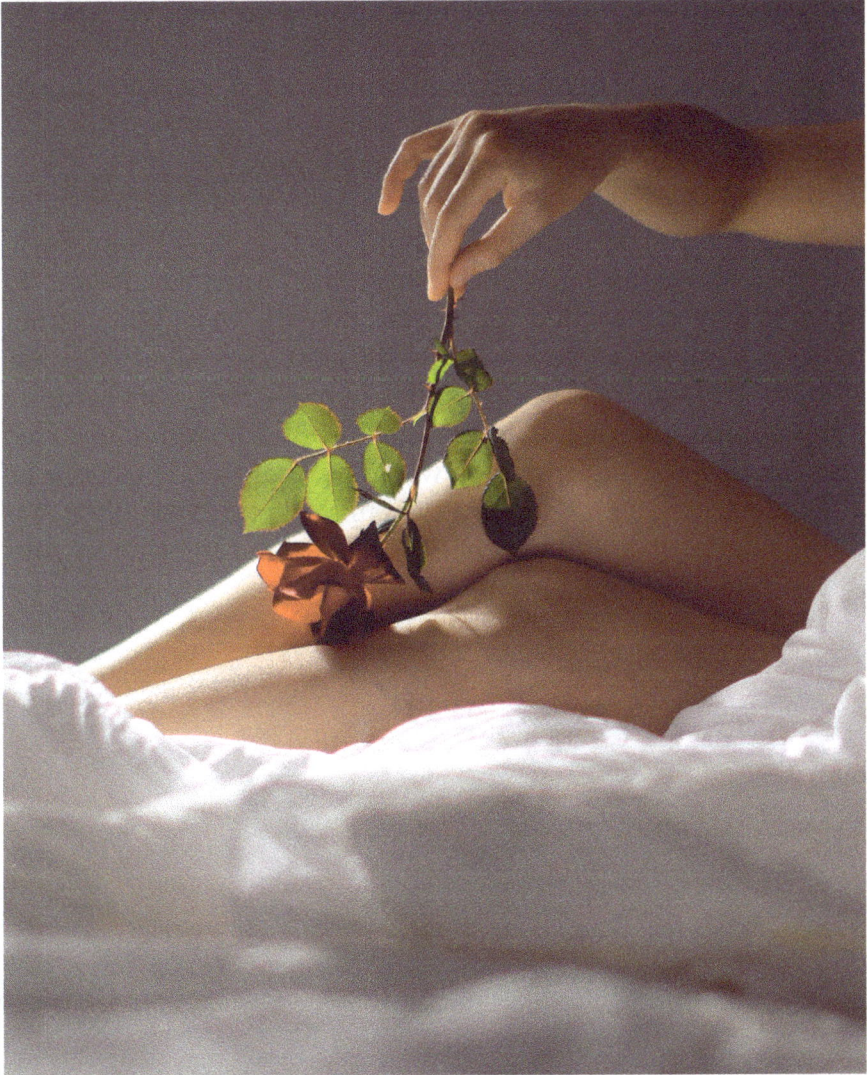

~ CHAPTER 7 ~

The sensual touch

With ordinary sex, tactile sensations are predominant, and the other four senses tend to take second place. It may sound odd, but most practices of tantric sex don't even require the subjects to use their hands to touch each other, but that won't obstacle in achieving great pleasure; instead, it exalts the fusion of the spirits.

Tantric sex isn't only a little influx of enjoyment but a profound and hypnotizing wave of pleasure brought by the orgasm. It's astounding how few changes applied in sex may take to different outcomes. Tantric sex doesn't generally involve much contact, nor does it need to consider making loud noises. Tantric sex is mainly based on using the balancing and expansion of internal energies to achieve absolute pleasure.

IMPORTANT: The massage techniques that I will explain to you next shouldn't be applied before the tantric sex. If you do so, you may get excited too soon, and you and your partner may get to an orgasm even before the actual sexual activity has started. The tantric massages that I am sharing with you are not a companion of the actual fusion but are techniques that you can use to build intimacy with your partner. These can be valid alternatives for a romantic evening to spend together, and they can give a sip of the benefits that Tantra can bring in your life and relationship.

7.1 HOW TO TOUCH YOUR SHIVA

In contrast to an ordinary sensual massage, the tantric massage of the penis and lingam it's not just meant to provoke your partner's physical orgasm. Instead, with this massage technique, you want to slowly awaken this critical erogenous zone and the powerful sexual energy hidden in it. Here's how to perform a tantric massage on your man.

First, it is essential to create a distraction-free environment where you can let yourself be absorbed entirely in the moment. For this reason, remove any irritating and disturbing element, i.e., clocks or any font of noise or undesired light. Another reason for eliminating clocks from the room is that this massage can take a long time. We are not interested in keeping track of time but only in the sensations we are experiencing at that moment. As suggested before, you can light up the room with scented candles and incense to make the atmosphere even more engaging.

Start the foreplay as you usually would, touch your partner until sexual arousal. Try to involve all the senses. Strip slowly to engage his sense of sight. Caress his body to engage the sense of touch. Let him feel the scent of your skin and the taste of your kisses. Bring him to arousal with words or moans of pleasure Before starting the authentic tantric massage, it is essential to know how your partner reacts to the stimulation of his different erogenous zones. Try to understand which are more sensitive and which are less, exploring not only the penis but also the perineum, the scrotum, and the inner thigh.

Oil is a fundamental element in Tantric massage. I recommend that you use sweet almond, coconut, or jojoba oil to enhance your sexual experience. Another essential element while performing the lingam (penis) massage is breathing. Both partners should use the *Bliss Breath* technique that consists of a series of deep breaths. First, inhale and focus on receiving the energy of arousal and pleasure from your partner. Then, exhale and focus on sending them loving energy. Continue to use this breathing technique during the massage.

Oil the shaft of the penis and the testicles. Start by slowly sliding your hands up and down the thighs. Wait until your partner feels relaxed and his body got used to your touch.

Move on the testicles. Gently, slowly massage them. Remember to keep using the Bliss Breath. Feel free to softly use your fingernails or slightly pull the testicles to provide some extra stimulation. During this massage, do not neglect the pubic bone in the front, the inner part of the thighs, and the perineum (the area between the testicles and the anus).

When you feel your partner aroused enough, start working on the shaft of the penis. During this process, it is essential to experiment with different approaches. Variety is the key to achieving the perfect orgasm. Here some ideas:

- Vary your grip from harder to lighter.
- Vary the speed from slow to fast. Then, you can tease your lover, building up from slow to fast and going back to slow again.
- Alternate strokes with one and two hands. Also, when you work with one hand, you can alternate left and right.
- Add some twisting in your strokes from time to time.
- Alternate deep strokes, that start from the base of the penis until the head, and short and rapid strokes.
- When playing with two hands, the bottom hand can move up and down while the top hand can add a twisting motion on the tip of the penis.

It is important not to let your partners come too quickly. Instead, try to keep him on the verge of orgasm. This is not an easy task; it requires some practice in reading his body language. Some indicators that an orgasm is imminent are changes in their breathing and involuntary micro muscle contractions. When you see them at the edge, pull back on what you are doing, or just slow it down and remind them to breathe and ride the wave of orgasmic feelings they are experiencing.

Start to stimulate the prostate (externally). To find the prostate (also called sacred spot), look for an indentation between the testicles and the anus. This spot has typically the size of a pea. Lightly press the area with your fingers or knuckles or use a circular massage motion. Let your partner guide you in order to apply the correct pressure. This spot is very sensitive. Try not to press too hard. Especially in the beginning, it is a good idea to ask your partner how they feel.

If your partner wants to try some anal play, you can stimulate the sacred spot internally. But, first, ensure that both your fingers and the area are well lubricated. Then, start massaging the outside of the anus in a slow circular motion. This will help loosen up the anal muscles making easy the penetration. Next, slowly insert the tip of your finger and move it until you feel minimal resistance. Remember to keep adding oil since the anus, unlike the vagina, is unable to lubricate itself. Once your partner feels comfortable, start to search for the prostate, usually situated 2 to 3 inches inside the anus, closer to the anterior wall of the rectum.

Once you reach the prostate, you can massage it moving your finger side to side or apply gentle pressure. Ask your partner how he feels so that you can adjust the movement based on how he feels.

To end the massage, you can allow your partner to climax or move on to sex.

7.2 How to Touch Your Shakti

One of the most famous tantric massages for ladies is the Yoni massage. If you have forgotten, the word *yoni* is the Sanskrit word used for the female genital organ.

Some allude to the vagina as a "consecrated sanctuary." This is because the vagina is an erogenous zone with the right to be investigated in an unexpected way, symbolizing the entrance to paradise.

Yoni has a primary role in Tantra. If you remember from the chapter describing the story of this sacred path, Tantra was born with the image of the female figure as its focus, and, of course, the vagina has the most crucial role in this part.

The fundamental objective of the Yoni massage is to make the lady profoundly excited and experience sensations that she has never experienced before. Also, the massage performed by men's fingers further expands the level of intimacy between the couple. The accomplice of the massage is classified "giver," to give the lady all the pleasure she merits and ought to anticipate nothing consequently.

Remember that I don't recommend using any of these massages before making love since these techniques accelerate the coming of the orgasm. If you decide to use this massage, you must consider that, if you do it properly, your female partner should reach the orgasm (and even having more than one), and you'll probably end without sex.

But, if you decide to try this massage, I am sure your lady will be very grateful. So, get ready to learn the Yoni massage procedure!

Set up the room. As mentioned in the previous chapters, be sure the light is right, and there are no distractions in the room.

The lady should lie on her back in a comfortable position with a pillow under her hips, the knees up, and the feet on the ground.

Synchronize your breathing. For the Yoni massage to work, it is significant that your breathing is synchronized. Try to inhale and exhale out together, keeping your breathing regular and slow. It is advisable to use the Bliss Breath; this technique consists of a series of deep breaths. First, inhale and focus on receiving the energy of arousal and pleasure from your partner. Then, exhale and focus on sending them loving energy. Continue to use this breathing technique during the massage.

Before starting with the real massage we want to do a short warm-up. Oil is a fundamental element; I recommend using sweet almond, coconut, or jojoba oil to enhance your sexual experience. Start to apply some oil on the belly and gently massage the area. Don't neglect the rib cage between the breasts and the lower abdomen. Use slow and delicate movements until you reach the breasts and the areolae. Don't touch the nipples yet until it is not clear that your lady is ready for it!

When you both think it is the right moment, start to tease the nipples alternating between circle movements and light pinching. Then, when you feel that your partner is aroused enough, it's time to perform the real yoni massage. You can apply various techniques to stimulate your partner; feel free to mix them based on your partner's feelings.

1. **Circles:** With this technique, we want to stimulate the external tip of the clitoris with a circular motion of the fingers. You can vary the pressure and the size of the circles based on your partner's reactions.
2. **Push & Pull:** Slide your finger down both sides of the shaft of the clitoris. Most people are more sensitive on one part of the clitoris than another; check your partner's reaction to understand where you should stimulate more.

3. **Tug & Roll:** You grasp the clitoris from the sides and gently pull back and forth with this technique. You can also gently roll the clitoris between your fingers.

4. **Tapping:** You can use one or more fingers to tap the clitoris gently.

5. **G-Spot Massage:** To find the G-Spot, curve your first two fingers like the letter "C" and slowly insert them in the vagina. About an inch or two in, you should feel a slightly ridged area at the top of the vaginal canal, just behind the external clitoris. Slowly stimulate that spot, first with gentle pressure or circle movements and later with a mix of fast and slow strokes.

Remember that the primary goal of Yoni massage is not having an orgasm; it is about feeling waves of pleasure ed eventually have multiple orgasms.

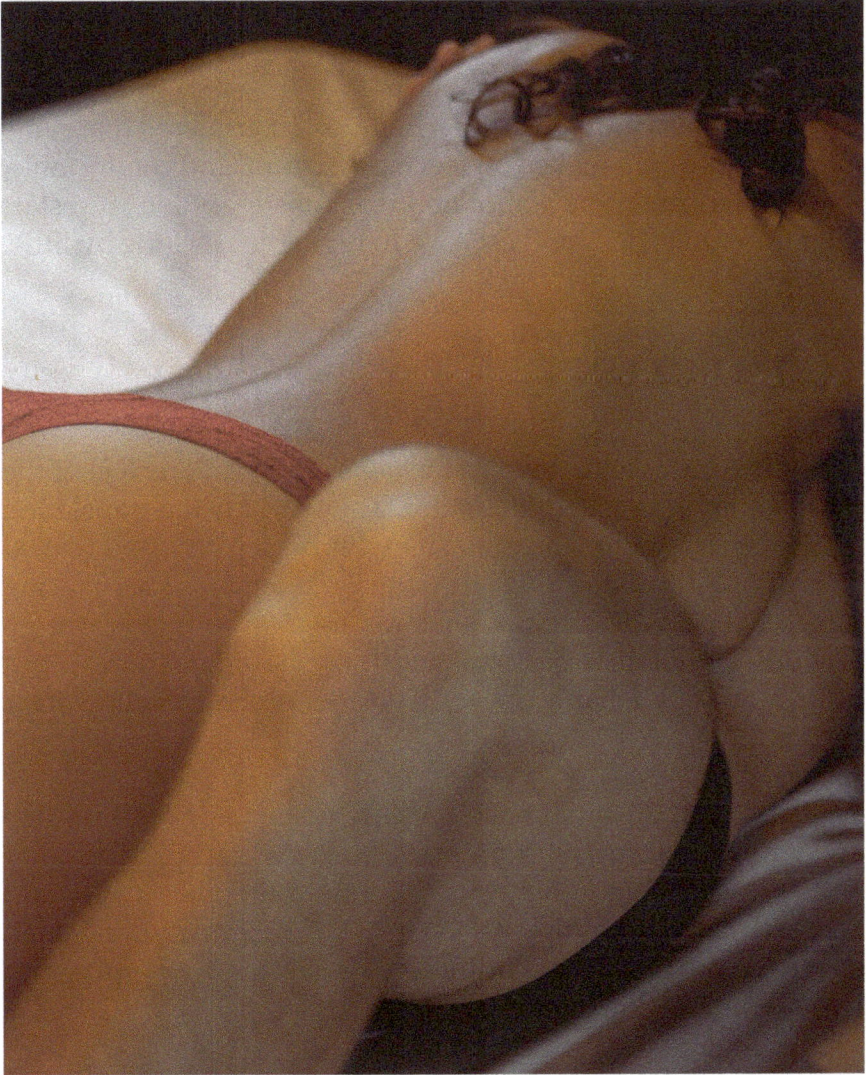

~ CHAPTER 8 ~

Tantric Positions

This chapter is probably the one you were waiting for and the reason you bought this book. Now that you have prepared your body and the environment to accomplish the tantric sex, it's time to know some positions that you can try with your partner.

For each technique, I added an indication of its difficulty in performing it. Still, you should consider that the complexity of one position depends on the strength and flexibility of the two subjects. So, finding a tantric position easy or complex is subjective to the couple.

Anyway, when I judged these techniques, I considered that some movements might make you feel more natural and comfortable, while others are more elaborated. So, my suggestion is to start with the easiest ones and escalate to higher levels little by little.

1. YAB YUN

The Yab Yum, even known as the *lotus sex position*, is one of the most common practices in Tantra. The world is the translation of "Father-Mother." The man sits with his legs crossed (called "Easy Pose"), and the lady sits on the gentleman's knees facing him, wrapping her legs around his torso. The hands can go around each other's back, or waist, or shoulders, or you can even move your hand on your partner's chest, feeling their beating.

You can reach this final position slowly, starting both from the "easy pose" (sitting with your legs crossed) facing each other and spending some time watching into each other's eyes and synchronizing your breaths. When you are ready, the lady slowly changes position sitting on his legs and wrapping her legs around his lower back.

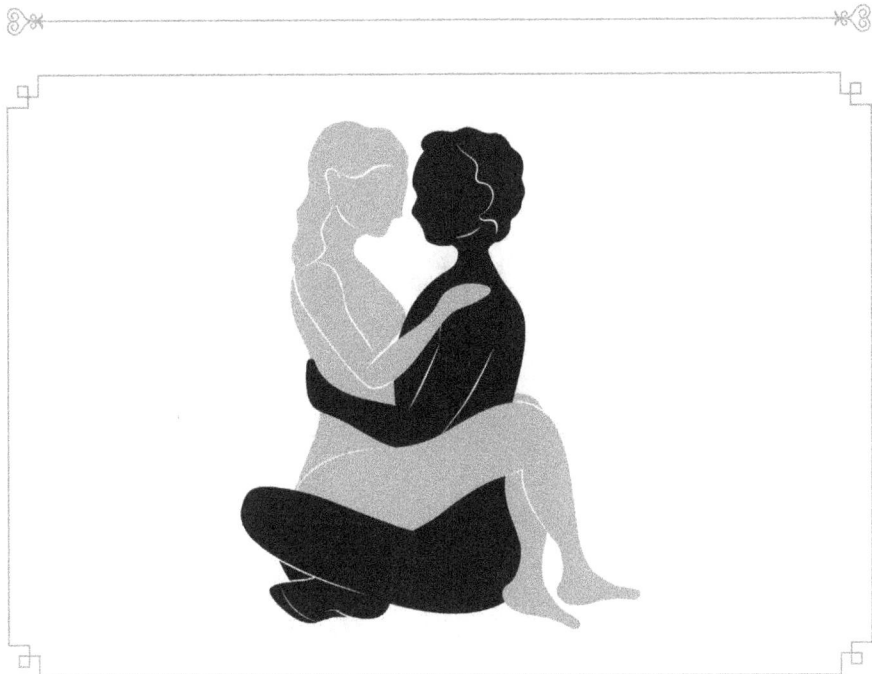

Complexity 🔥🔥🔥🔥🔥

While executing the Yab Yum position, you can close your eyes since you are supposed to keep the connection with your partner through the touch and synchronization of your breaths.

In this position, you should feel your bodies exchanging energy. The female power (and the creative life force) rises while the man sits under the woman giving his support as a solid container. Two opposite forces united into one shape.

Hint: Usually, the men don't resist staying in the easy pose for long. You can use some pillows to make him feel more comfortable. He can sit on them or use them under his knees.

2. Sidewinder (Side wind-her)

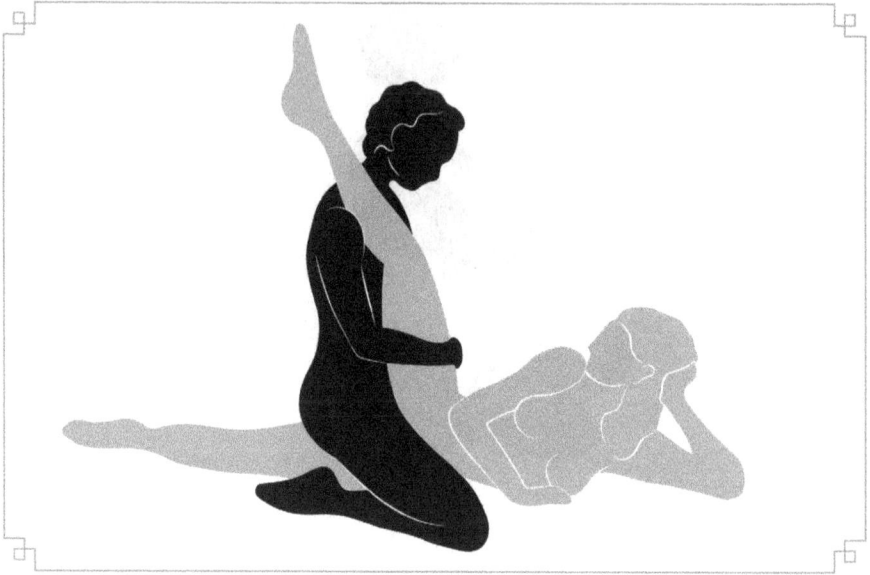

Complexity 🔥 🔥 🔥 🔥 🔥

The girl should lie on one side and raise the top leg, keeping the bottom one straight on the floor. The gentleman should sit on the bottom lady's thigh, hugging the extended leg on the top; the lady's caff resting on his shoulder.

Hint: Once he is inside her, the man should whirl his hips as he thrusts. With these movements, he'll be able to touch different zones inside the woman's vagina, raising the pleasure to a higher level.

3. PADLOCK

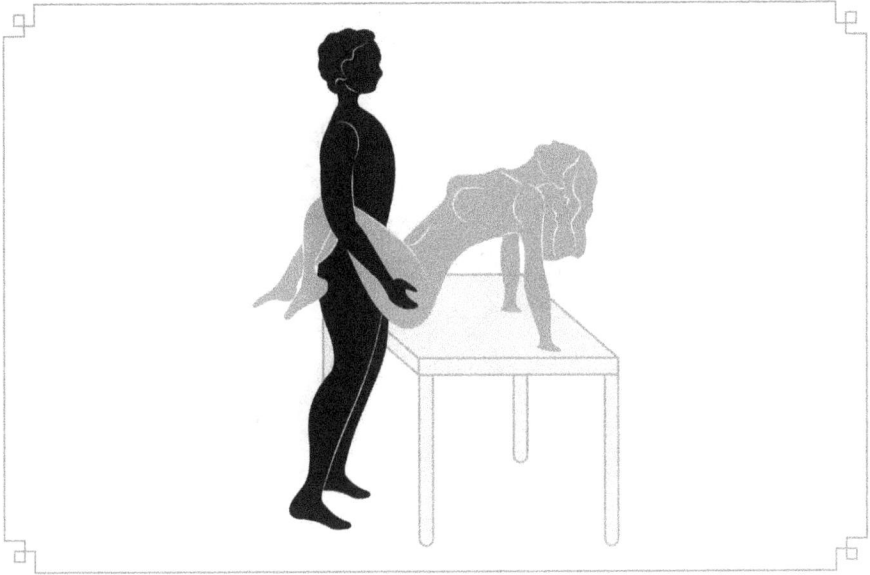

Complexity 🔥 🔥 💧 💧 💧

In this position, the girl sits at the edge of a waist-high piece of furniture, opening her legs and using her arms to support her upper body. Then, the man comes in between the lady's legs, penetrating her, and she wraps her legs around him. For this final shape, this position is also known as *Leg Lock*. Tables and washing machines suit perfectly for this performance. If the man needs added height, he can use some support to stand on it. This position makes it easy for the penetrating partner to stimulate the woman's clitoris.

Hint: With this technique, it's easy for you to keep eye contact. Start this by looking into each other's eyes to increase your affinity, but when it comes, feel free to close your eyes and get lost in the pleasure.

4. Amazing Butterfly

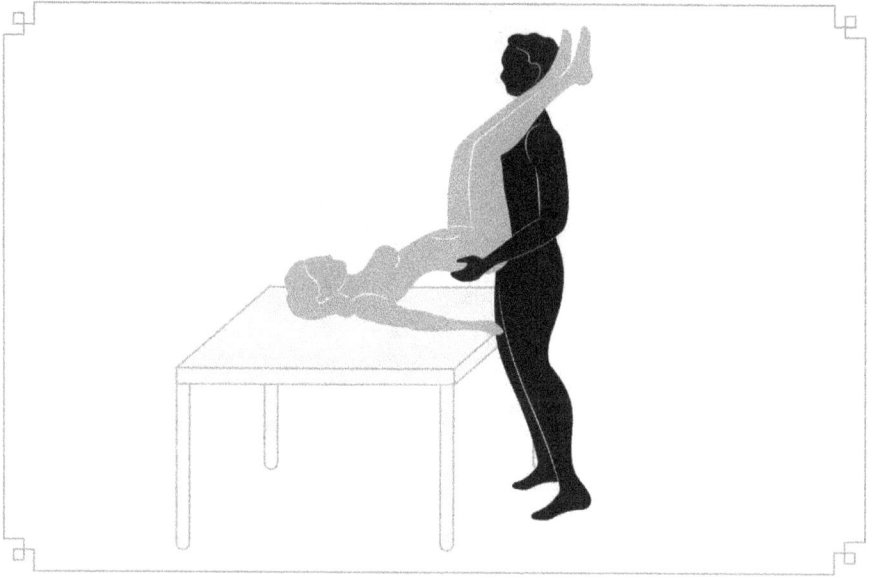

Complexity 🔥🔥🔥🔥🔥

Starting from the padlock position, you can make things a little more challenging. First, the girl should lie on the table and raising her legs, resting her calves on the partner's shoulders. Next, the man should support the lady's back, placing his hands under her hips. With this position, the booty is at the perfect angle while he thrusts.

Hint: In this position, the pelvic tilt gives his penis full access to the vagina exposing female zones that are very sensitive to pleasure. The man should make slow movements and try different pressures to explore what his lady likes most.

5. MERMAID

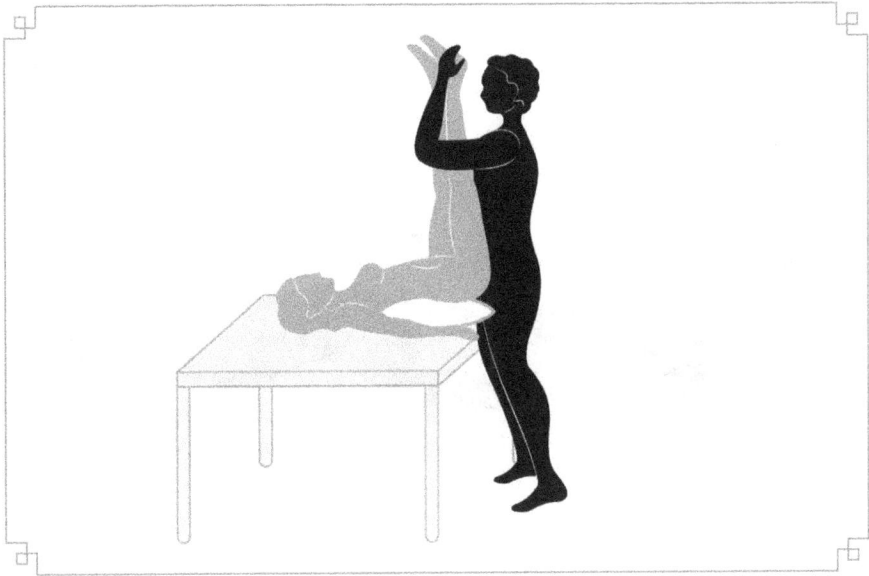

Complexity 🔥🔥🔥🔥🔥

The Mermaid position is another technique that requires medium-high. Very similar to the previous two, the lady lies on her back and raises her legs. But, in the earlier positions, the legs were widely spread apart. For this technique, they need to stay together, like having a long fishtail instead of two legs (which explains the name of this pose).

Hint: To make the Mermaid position more comfortable, make sure that you and your partner's genital are almost at the same level to facilitate the penetration. Also, to avoid reducing his mobility and comfort, the man should avoid bending his knees; instead, he should stand straight. Finally, remember that he can acquire some extra-high using some support if needed.

6. Double Decker

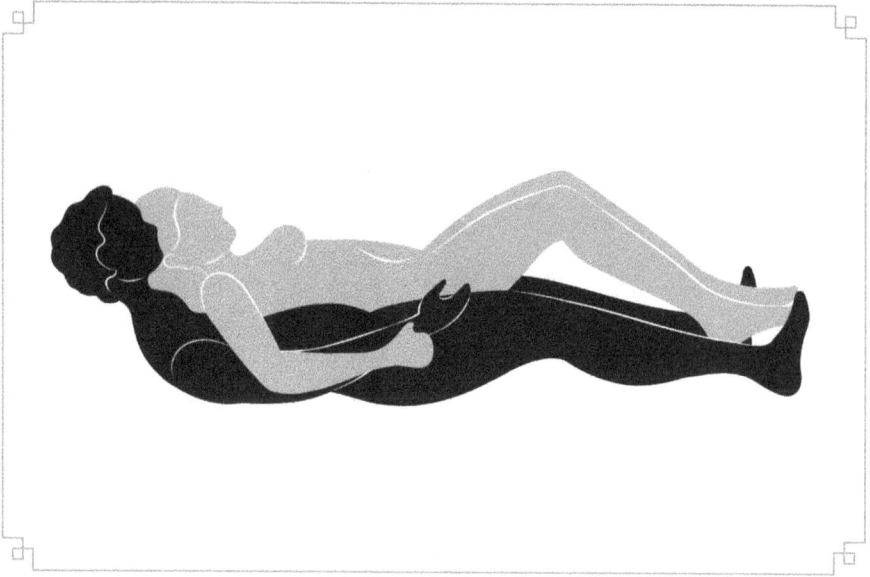

Complexity 🔥🔥🔥🔥🔥

This position's name comes probably from the popular double-decker buses that became an icon for London, England. During the Double Decker, the two partners lie on their backs, having the lady on top of him. The receiving partner's back on the giver's chest while he penetrates her from behind. Tantric sex rarely allows the men to lie on their back, but this position is an exception since the G-Spot is easy to reach because perfectly aligned with the angle of penetration.

Hint: You can decide to use this technique to penetrate the anus instead of the vagina. In this way, you can try this position with two different variations. For this reason, the Double Decker is recommended for gay or lesbian couples too.

7. Lap Dance

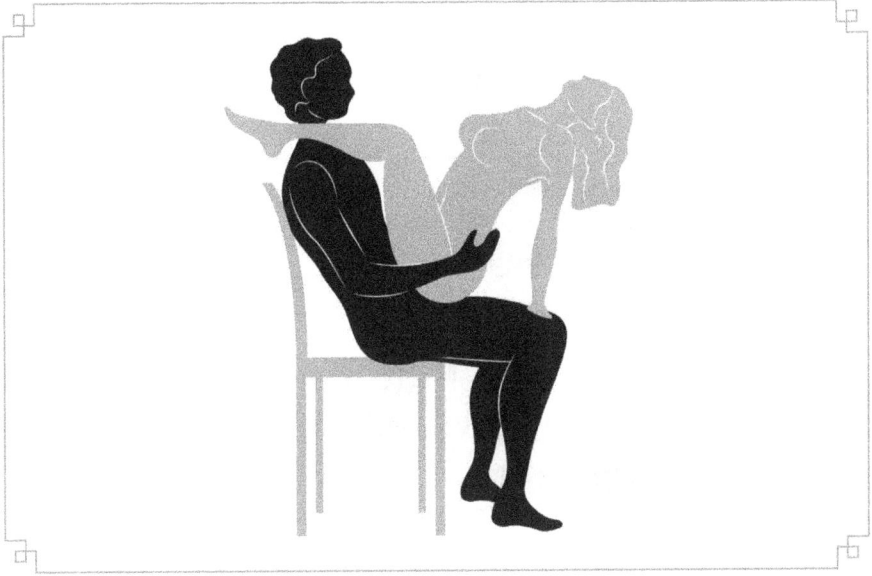

Complexity 🔥 🔥 🔥 🔥 🔥

The Lap Dance position is a technique where the woman mainly controls the sexual activity while the man can choose to relax and 'enjoy the show' or be a bit more proactive. To perform it, the man must sit on a chair or sofa with the legs wide open. Next, the girl sits on him, guiding his member into the vagina. Then, she should lean backward slightly, placing her hands on his knees. Finally, the lady's legs should extend, resting the ankles on his shoulders.

Hint: To improve the thrusting power, the lady can adjust the weight between the ankles and the hands. The man should tilt his back a little for a better connection, using an angle between 100° and 120° instead of straight at 90°. Also, he can use a pillow to feel more comfortable.

8. G-Force

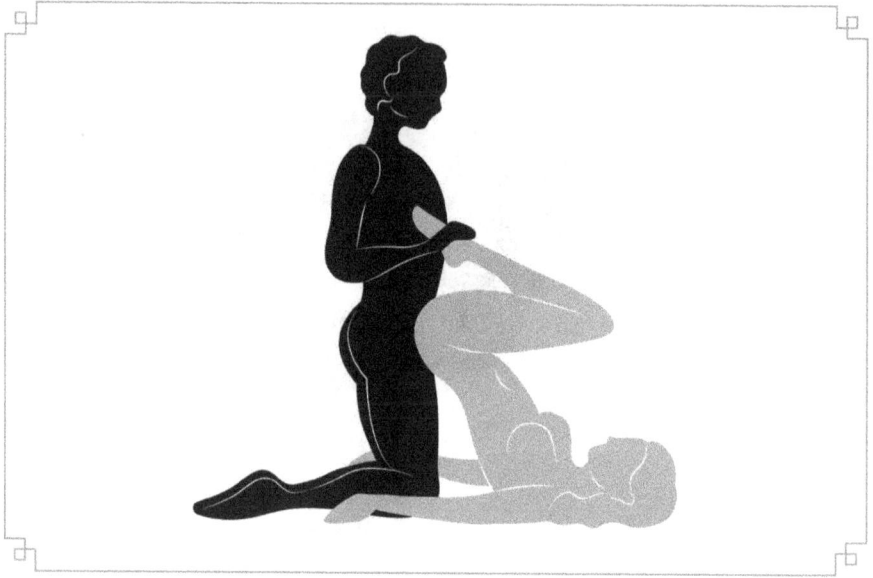

Complexity 🔥🔥🔥🔥🔥

The girl lies down on her back and pulls the knees close to her chest to start this position. Next, the man kneels, pulling her from her hips when penetrating her. Once the partners are connected, the man can move his hands to grab her feet and penetrate. This position is perfect to stimulate her G-Spot and allows the man to be in control. G-Force also allows a reasonable degree of eye contact, and the mane can enjoy the lady's expressions while giving her pleasure.

Hint: For a variation of this position, the lady can place her calves on his shoulders. This new angle of penetration will change the zones stimulated inside her vagina, giving her a new gamma of sensations.

9. WATERFALL

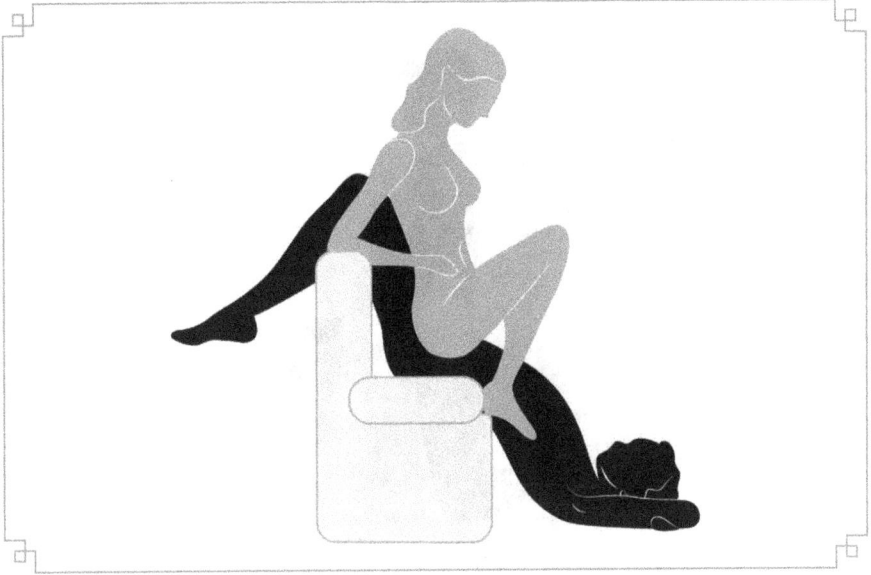

Complexity 🔥🔥🔥🔥🔥

In the Waterfall is a position the woman is on top. The man lies face up with the head and torso off the edge of the bed and the shoulders resting on the ground. The lady sits then on top of, him leading the penetration. With this technique, the receiving partner is in control, and from her point of view, she can see the companion's reaction. In addition, the blood floating to the head of the gentleman will amplify his sensations.

Hint: You can try this position on the sofa or the armchair, with the giver's legs resting on the backrest.

10. PASSION PRETZELL

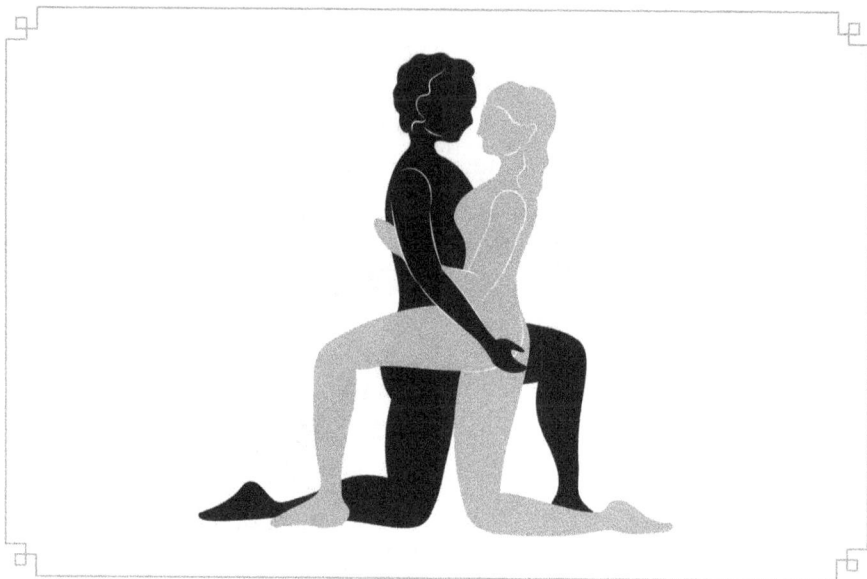

Complexity 🔥 🔥 🔥 🔥 🔥

In this position, you are both kneeling, facing each other. Both of you should place the opposite foot flat on the ground and get closer until penetrating. Then, you and your partner should alternate in leaning forward and backward for thrusting, keeping your lower parts planted to the floor. With this position, male and female roles are equal, two opposite parts completing each other. Use your free arms and hands to build up more intimacy, and remember to keep eye contact.

Hint: It's challenging to maintain this position for a long time; remember to stay as comfortable as possible performing it on a carpet and using pillows. If you start to struggle, consider transitioning into the Yab Yum position to release the tension in your muscles.

11. TUB TANGLE

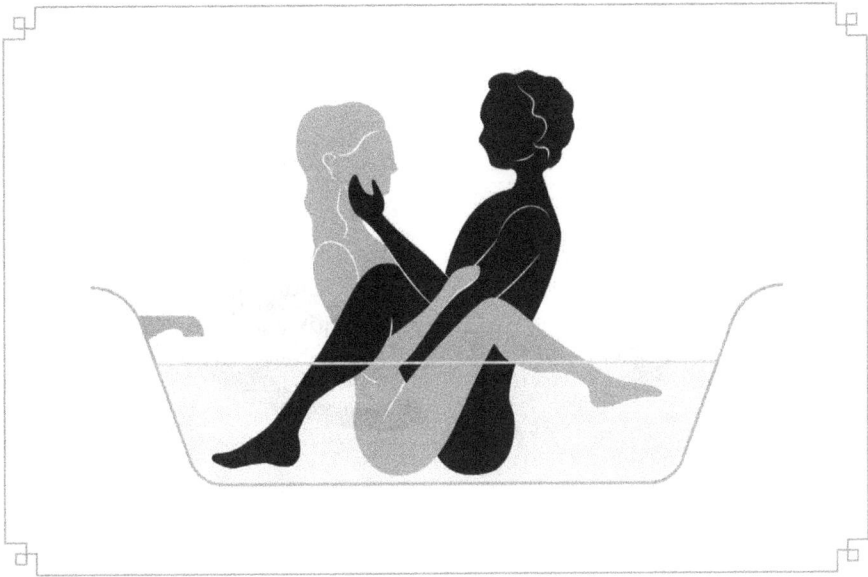

Complexity 🔥🔥🔥🔥🔥

What I love about tantric sex is how your surroundings can help to experiment with some techniques, so most of the rooms in the house can be inspiring for trying different experiences. This position is the one to try in the bathtub, facing each other and both of you with the knees bent, keeping the feet planted on the bottom of the bathtub. Once you get into contact, feel free to wrap the legs around your partner's back and link the elbows under each other's knees.

Hint: Since your lips are very close to each other, take this opportunity to exchange passionate kisses and play with your mouths.

12. Torrid Tidal Wave

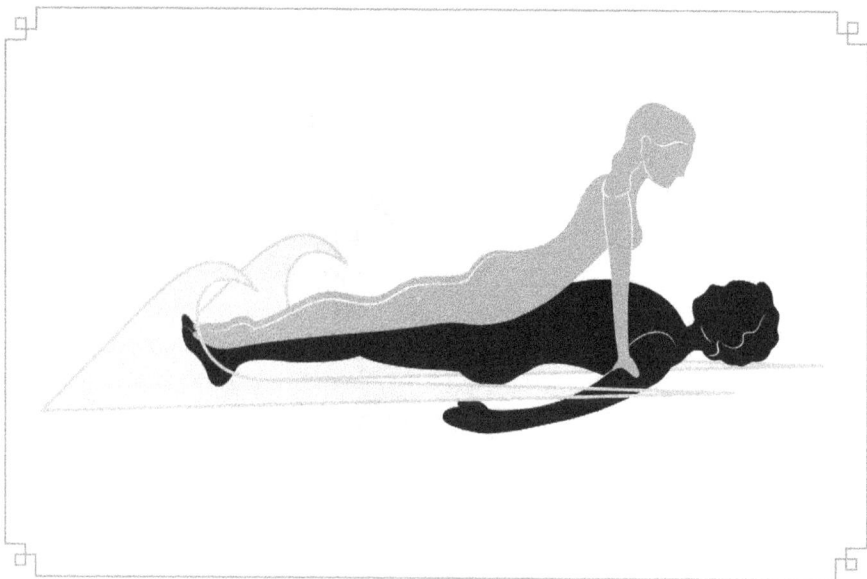

Complexity 🔥🔥🔥🔥🔥

The Torrid Tidal Wave is the perfect position to try during a vacation and make you feel like two teenagers. The man lies on his back at the water's edge on a beach, keeping the legs extended and together. The woman lays face-down on him, having the pelvises aligned. Then the lady expands her arms to lift her torso, putting her weight on the hands. In this position, enjoy the waves on your skin; they will amplify your sensations.

Hint: With this technique, the clitoris rubs against the man's pelvic bone. The lady should sporadically clench her butt cheeks tight to increase the feeling of the penis inside her body.

13. Great Bee

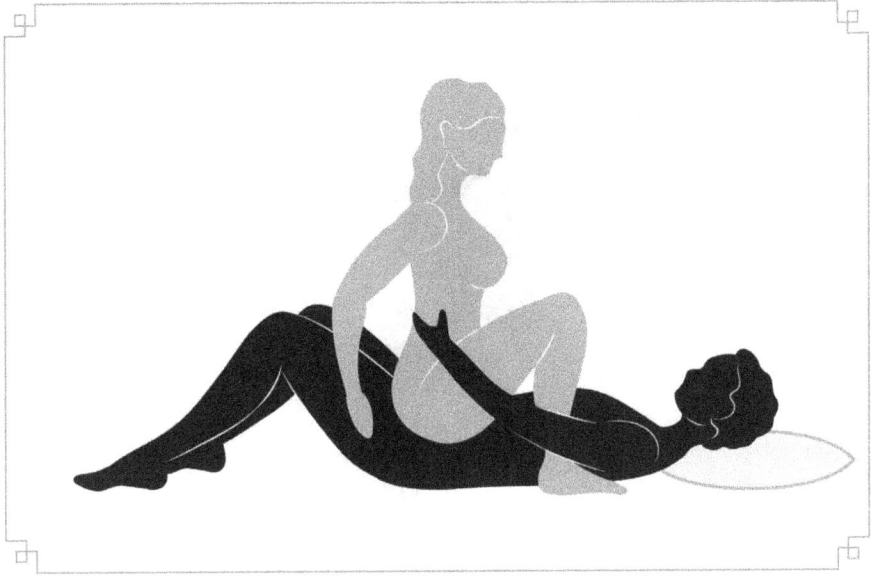

Complexity 🔥🔥🔥🔥🔥

For the Great Bee, the man lies down on his back while the lady sits on him in a squat position, having her knees blended to her chest. In this situation, she has absolute control of the tantric sex. Supporting herself with her hands against the lover's thighs, she can perform every movement that she wants, controlling the speed, the penetration, and the frequency.

Hint: When thrusting, I suggest the lady rotate her hips in wide circles. Try also with different pressures on his body to make him feel different intensities.

14. Time Bomb

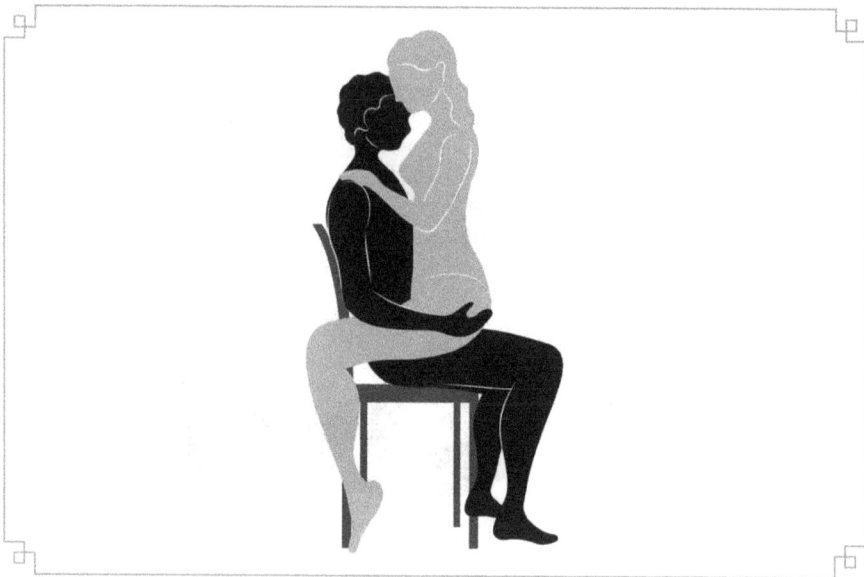

Complexity 🔥🔥🔥🔥🔥

In the Time Bomb, the man is sitting on a chair, having his legs relaxed. The woman approaches, facing him and sitting on his erected member; her legs loosened too, having the feet reaching the floor. The arms of both are free, so you can use them to increase your intimacy, like having your hands on each other's chests to adjust your breaths.

Hint: In this position, the woman is in control. When penetrating, do it slowly, inch by inch, to the very end. Then increase the speed gradually to make him feel the different sensations.

15. LOVE TRIANGLE

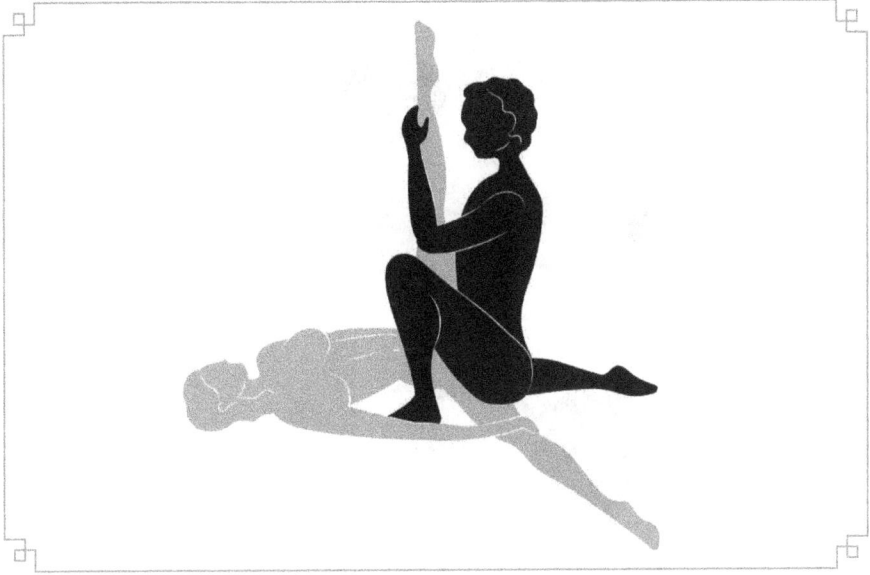

Complexity 🔥 🔥 🔥 🔥 🔥

In the Love Triangle position, the woman lies on her back with the left leg sticking on the floor while the right one is straight up in the air. Having her helping herself with the right hand under the knee, she should stretch her right leg on the side, having it at 90° to her body. If you are akin to geometry, this shape reminds the z-axis in a 3D cartesian coordinate system. Once she is in position, the male partner should crouch at the bottom of her body and start penetrating.

Hint: From this position, the man has free access to the whole vagina. When penetrating, he can rotate his body slightly to try different angulations.

16. One Pincer

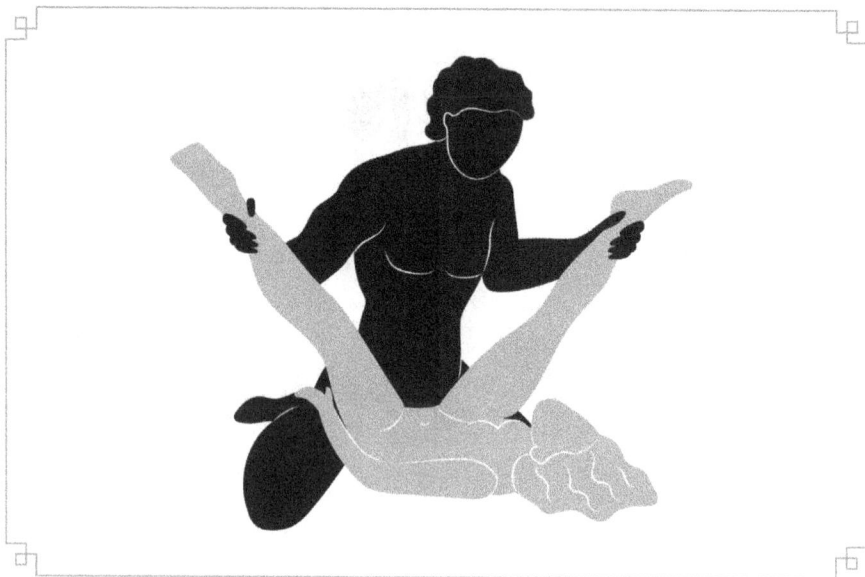

Complexity 🔥 🔥 🔥 🔥 🔥

The lady lies down on her back with the legs spread wide open in the One Pincer position. The partner kneels in front of her, grabbing her feet and supporting her legs. In this sex experience, the man is in control, but the lady can have some authority too from her bottom position. She can use her free arms to pull the partner's tights to her body, suggesting the speed of the penetration.

Hint: With this position, the man not only can access the vagina freely, but he has free access to the anus as well, in case you want to try this experience too.

17. TILTED MISSIONARY

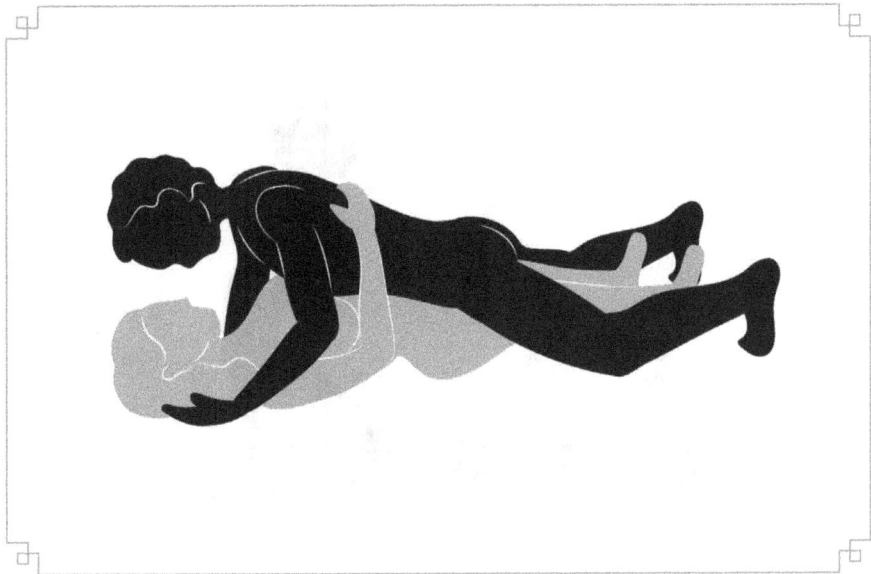

Complexity 🔥 🔥 🔥 🔥 🔥

There is a reason why some positions are more famous than others. The different techniques that you can apply with the missionary pose allow a better connection between the couple and keep the upper body free enough to build synchronization and look into each other eyes. The lady lies on her back while the man lies on top of her facing each other. For a more comfortable position, the woman can add a pillow under her butt; this will also help to have the vagina more exposed.

Hint: After some time in this position, I suggest the lady moving her legs over the man's shoulders. With this variation, the penetrating part can reach the G-Spot easily and experience some jolts of great pleasure.

18. SNAKE TRAP

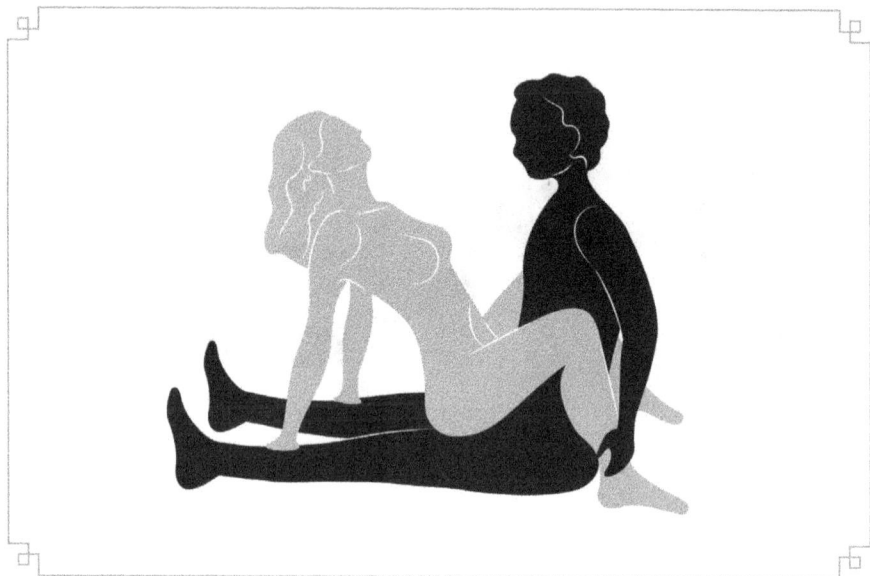

Complexity 🔥🔥🔥🔥🔥

The Snake Trap position should be performed in bed or on the floor. The man sits down with his torso straight, and the legs open in a V shape. The lady approaches facing him and sits on him, having the legs in the same shape as the male partner's. The couple is now sitting across from one another, facing each other. The torso should lean backward slightly for both the accomplices, supporting the weight on their hands.

Hint: This position is for shallow penetrations. For better stabilization, grab your partner's ankles, and adjust your torso.

19. SPOONING SEX

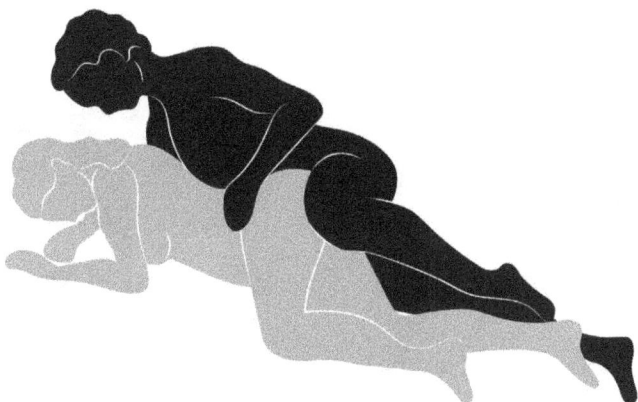

Complexity 🔥🔥🔥🤍🤍

You may already know this technique for cuddling. The two partners are lying down on their side, the butt of the woman in contact with his genitals. They look like two spoons positioned side by side, and this explains the name. To adjust this position for tantric sex, the lady lies on one side with the knees a bit bent, while the male partner lies on her upper side coming from the back. For the penetration, her legs should open a bit more to allow him to access, and then you can adjust the position once you are connected, making yourselves comfortable. Since the giver partner is coming from the back, this technique is ideal for stimulating her G-Spot. You can try this position also for anal sex.

Hint: Make use of your free arms to cuddling each other. With this position, the giver can kiss his partner's neck and ear if she likes it.

20. Serpent's Embrace

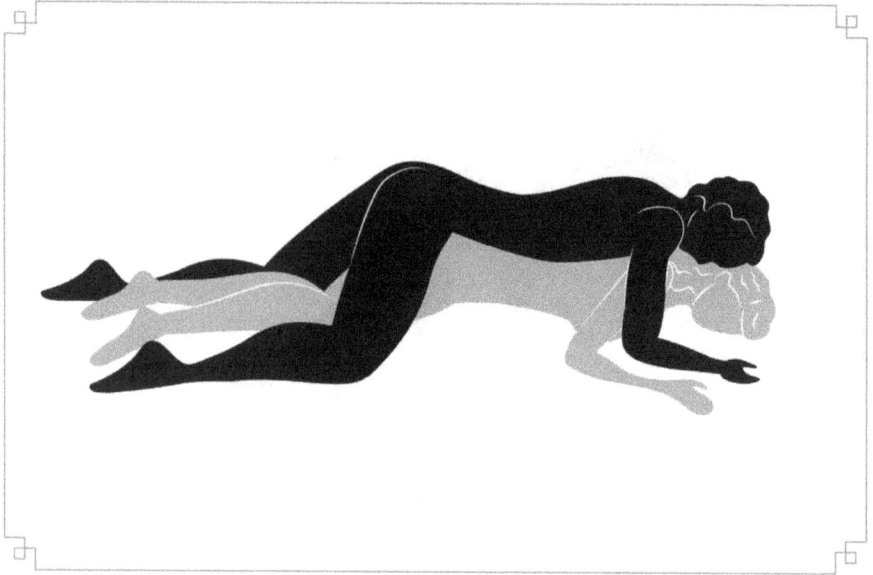

Complexity 🔥🔥🔥🔥🔥

This position reminds the spooning one, but instead of being on the side, the woman lies face-down, with a pillow under her hips to raise them a bit. Her forearms are planted on the ground to support her upper body and prop it up slightly. The male partner lies face-down on top of the lady, penetrating her from the back.

Hint: After some time in this position, I suggest the lady moving her legs over the man's shoulders. With this variation, the penetrating part can reach the G-Spot easily and experience some jolts of great pleasure.

21. Row His Boat

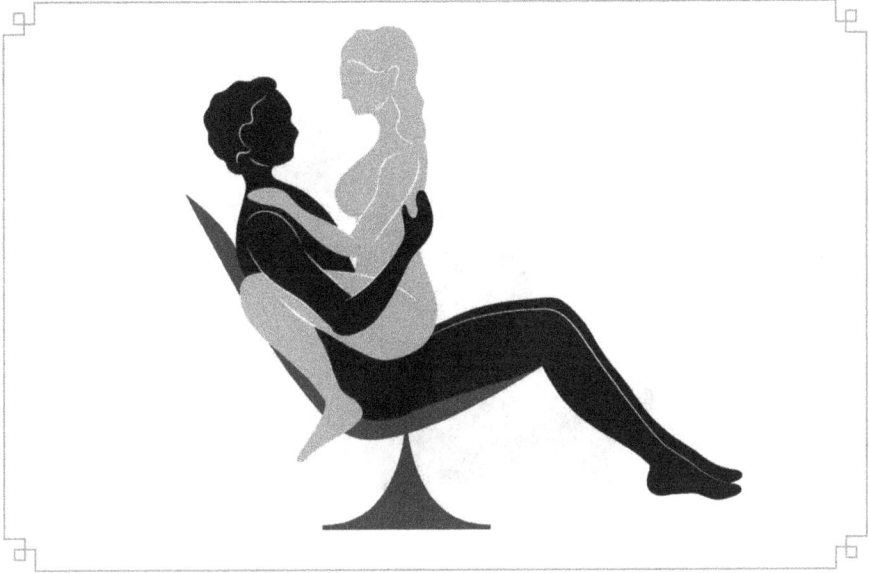

Complexity 🔥 🔥 🔥 🔥 🔥

For this position, the male part sits on a chair or sofa with the legs slightly spread. The lady sits on him, straddling his lap and facing him. Her legs are bent and open, passing under his arms, and the feet should lend against the seat of the chair. In this technique, the woman rides him, and she is in charge of the sexual activity. You can use your free arms for cuddling a little; your faces are also pretty close to each other so that you can exchange sweet kisses on the lips. During the waiving, the girl should try with different paces. Another suggestion is to make wide circular movements when thrusting.

Hint: The secret for this position is, for the man, to don't sit straight but to lean back a little. Try this position on a reclining chair to feel more comfortable.

22. WOW-HIM POWWOW

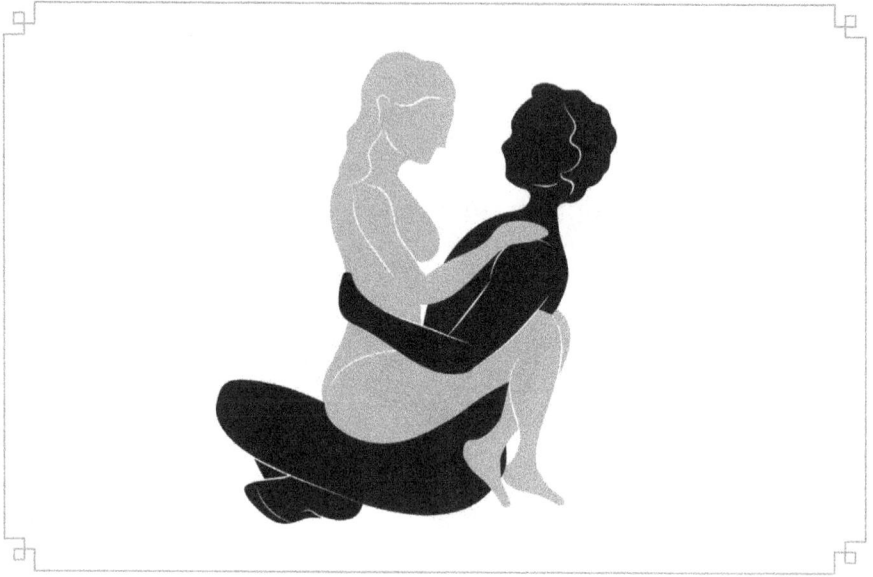

Complexity 🔥 🔥 🔥 🔥 🔥

This position is a slight variation of the Yan Yum. First, the man sits down with crossed legs while the lady sits on his lap facing him, leading his penis inside her vagina when sitting. Later, she wraps her legs around his torso while he leans backward a little. Then, holding each other's backs tightly, the couple should start to wave back and forth together, increasing the speed while getting used to the movement.

Hint: Change the way you move to try different levels of intimacy. You can speed up or slow down, get deep, or having shallow penetrations. Try different combinations find the combo that you like most.

23. Sofa Spread-Eagle

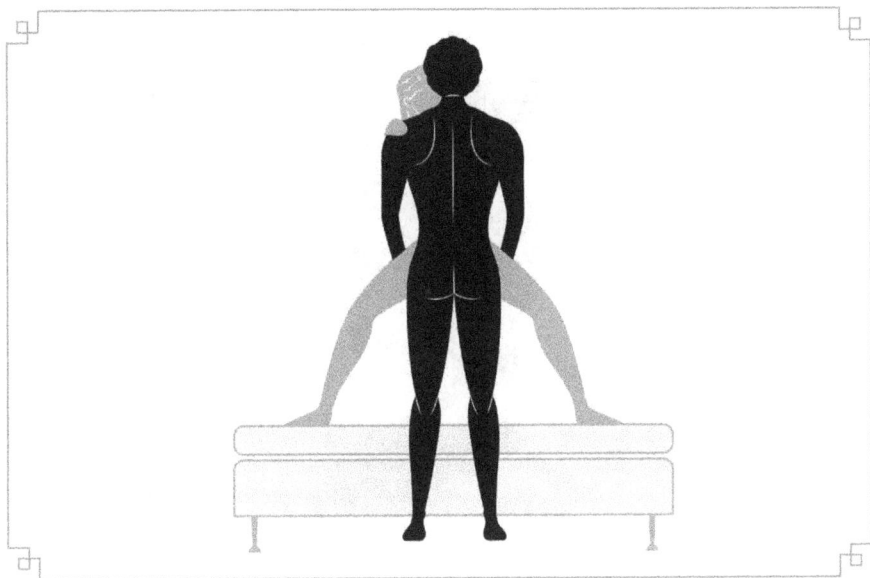

Complexity 🔥 🔥 🔥 🔥 🔥

The lady stands on the edge of a sofa or bed, with her legs spread wide. The man approaches her from the front, standing on the floor. The girl should adjust the height of her stance, extending the legs and bending her knees, while the man should stand straight.

Hint: The pelvises should be at the same level. If she is in a too high position, the man can help by adding some extra height under his feet.

24. HOT SEAT

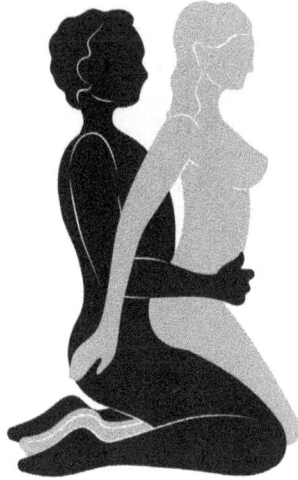

Complexity 🔥 🔥 🔥 🔥 🔥

The Hot Seat reminds the Yab Yun with the couple facing in the same direction instead of staring at each other. The male part kneels behind the girl, but he has to lean slightly backward. The lady kneels in front of him with the legs between his legs. Her back is touching his front part, and the bodies are squeezed together tightly. The giver's arms can go around her waist, while her hands can grab his forearms or hips. Once connected, try different depths, pressure, and speed.

Hint: When the giver is coming from the back, it's easier for the male member to touch the female G-Spot. The girl should try to swivel her hips in circular motions to stimulate this magic area even better.

25. Get Down On It

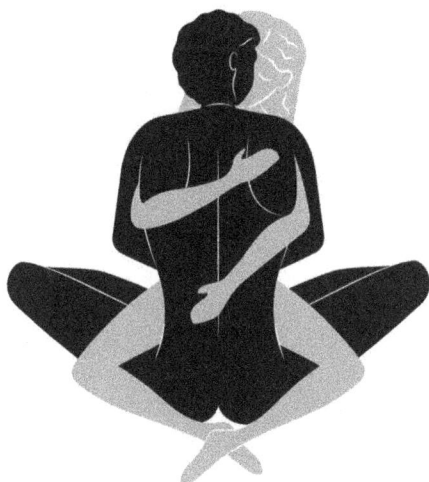

Complexity 🔥 🔥 🔥 🔥 🔥

This position is basically like the Yan Yum with some extra techniques helping with the synchronization between you and your partner. The man sits in the easy pose (with his legs crossed), and the woman sits on him, facing him and wrapping her legs around his waist. They should embrace each other and alternate their breaths, so when one inhales, the other exhales and vice versa. As the lady breathes in, rock your pelvis back and tighten the vaginal muscles. When she exhales, tilt the pelvis forward and release. The two parts should mirror each other.

Hint: Yoga fanatics would probably love this position since it helps with the perfect synchronization between the two lovers. For better intimacy, close your eyes and stay focus on your partner's breath. Don't rush to the waving; try to manage the mirroring of the breath first, and once you get used to it, you can apply the movements. The secret of this technique is to take it slow and relax.

CHAPTER 9

Orgasm

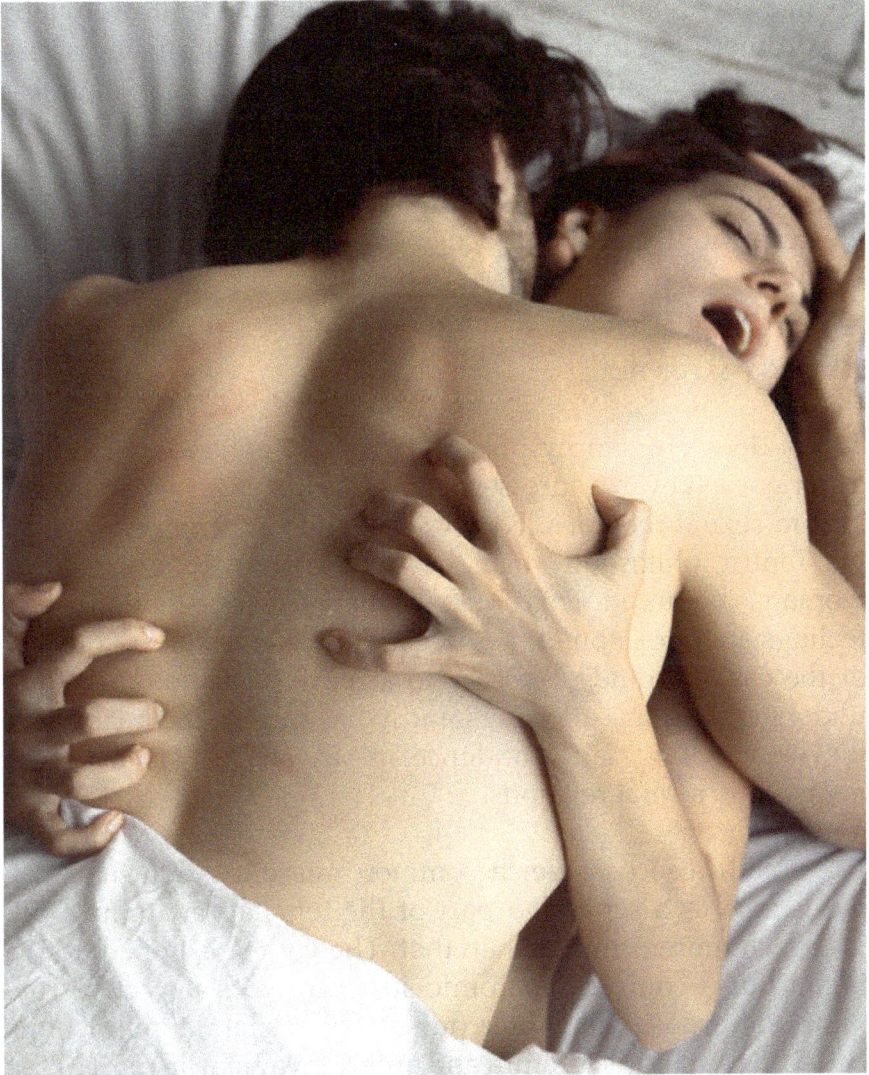

As most people probably already know, an orgasm is a sexual climax. The word orgasm is based on a Greek term meaning "to swell." In Tantra, orgasm is seen as a spiritual experience. But in following the Tantric tradition of slow lovemaking, the goal is generally to prolong orgasm as long as possible.

Many people are getting into Tantra in the last decade to add some fun into their relationship or overcome some issues when making love. Either way, Tantra approaches the experience of sex in a way that makes it supreme and unique. Unfortunately, the ordinary life in the society where we live is causing stress and disorder in our system, and these problems may manifest during sex, blocking us from the satisfaction that we deserve.

Tantric orgasm is about rejecting judgment and breathing into the moment. It's all about focusing the enrgies to finally realise them.

9.1 Orgasm for her

Tantra does not simply provide a way to enhance the sexual experience; it even addresses women's challenges when taking part in sexual relations. For example, it is a common belief in the Tantric philosophy that the most crucial sex organ for a woman is her mind. This organ is where negative thoughts and feelings are born, sometimes negatively affecting sexual desire or the ease of mind necessary to achieve pleasure. Therefore, understanding these feelings and what caused them can help the woman find self-confidence in sex and make her more involved in sexual relations.

We should also consider a common misconception that sees the vagina as a separated part of the female's anatomy. Still, it's much more complex than that. The vagina is not a passive organ but a complex anatomic structure with an active role in sexual arousal and intercourse. The dynamic interactions between the clitoris, urethra and anterior vaginal are part of the same complex clitourethrovaginal (CUV) system. This complex structure covers a large multifaceted morphofunctional area that, when properly stimulated, could bring to the big O. Here a few techniques that will help a woman in achieving a fantastic orgasm.

Explosive orgasm and implosive orgasm

A woman's orgasmic experience involves multiple erogenous zones in a hard-to-describe mix of sensations. Therefore, it is difficult to classify the various types of orgasms in their various facets. Still, we can use two macro-categories:

- **Explosive orgasm:** It can be represented by a powerful emanation of energy outside the woman's body.
- **Implosive orgasm:** Aims to a greater form of satisfaction.

The **explosive orgasm** involves the genital area and the lower chakras (the Base Chakra - the first - and the Sacral chakra - the second). These orgasms frequently leave a sense of fatigue and disappointment since it does not lead to the total satisfaction of mind and body. Clitoral orgasm is of this kind.

The **implosive orgasm** is an experience in which the energy doesn't scatter outside but collapses inwards, involving the upper chakras. It can include the entire body, just as the psychological and passionate circles of the lady, conveying a general sense of satisfaction and contentment. These types of orgasms are both physical and mental. The vaginal orgasm and the cervical-uterine orgasm are of this sort.

Clitoral Stimulation

Believe it or not, but there are ways for a woman to reach orgasm without passing through the penetration phase. In fact, according to a 2017 study, only about 18 percent of women achieve orgasm through penetration. Clitoral stimulation is beneficial when it comes to orgasming during sex. I mentioned before how the clitoris is such a receptive spot that it is even more sensitive than the men's penis. Of course, sex, in itself, is a critical stimulating demonstration; anyway, the clitoris is the pearl that gives the vast majority of the sexual joy that a woman experiences. For this reason, it is essential to focus on this area as much as possible before and during sex. It is important to be as gentle as possible when stimulating this area due to its incredible sensitivity.

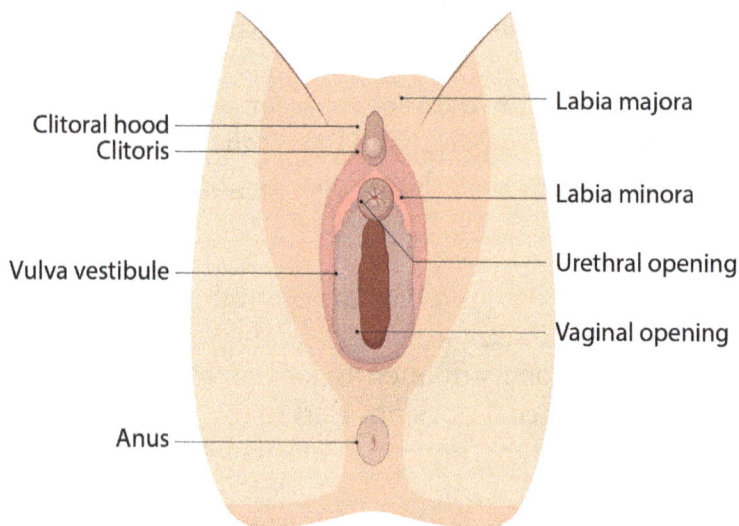

G-Spot

The exercises of Tantra show that there is a holy spot inside a woman's vagina called G-Spot, which is extremely sensitive. If stimulated correctly, this area can convey high peaks of pleasure for a woman. The "G" of the G-spot comes from Gräfenberg, a German physician and scientist who invented an intra-uterine device for his studies about female orgasm. His experiments revealed that there is a particular area inside the female reproductive system that produces intense stimulus. This spot can be easily found when performing the "come here" motion with the middle finger inside the vagina.

However, recent studies clarify that the G-Spot isn't a separated area of women's anatomy, but it's part of the clitoral network. So, stimulating the G-Spot is like stimulating the clitoris from the inside. Turns out, the little nub coming out where the inner labia meet is only the tip of the clitoris. Even if this magic area can be spotted with the "come here" motion of your finger, consider that this region varies from woman to woman, so there are cases where it's challenging to find the correct position. Anyway, it's worth it for a woman to explore her body and to locate her G-spot because once discovered, sex will move to much higher levels.

Cervical-uterine Orgasm

The cervical-uterine orgasm is much less famous than the clitoral and G-spot ones because it's not as common as the previous two, and it's not straightforward to recognize it. The cervix is a cylinder-shaped neck of tissue that connects the vagina and uterus. So to get to the cervix, it's going to involve deep penetration.

The area surrounded by the cervix presents many nerves distributed throughout the entire pelvis, so pressing this area or rubbing against it may bring the woman to an intense sense of pleasure.

Aiming for a cervical orgasm is not a simple thing; as said, the cervix is in a pretty deep position, then you may require a relatively long member to reach it. Also, each vagina has a different design, so you may need a particular angle or curve to get to the right spot.

If you want to try this experience, it may be an exciting journey to try also with your partner, especially if you are keen to attempt new experiments in bed. Most of the positions coming from behind are ideal for exploring the cervix zone; also, you may consider using a toy to amplify your research.

9.2 ORGASM FOR HIM

It is customary to believe that, for men, the orgasm manifests through ejaculation. Achieving this status is indeed the result of great pleasure. Still, the feeling of ecstasy usually lasts just a few moments before it gradually disappears and what follows is the lowest condition of sexual excitement for a man. After the peak, the man usually loses his interest, and he needs to wait some time before reactivating his sexual desire. For this reason, ejaculation is usually the end of lovemaking, which, on some occasions, may leave the woman not fully satisfied.

If you are a man, I know what you may be thinking: "How can I last longer? How can I limit my pleasure and delay my final orgasm?" Before answering it, I want to raise something that most people usually forget. Ejaculation and orgasm are two different things. Indeed you can have an orgasm that manifests through ejaculation, but they don't have necessarily come together.

In the end, orgasm is something happening in your mind. It's the feeling of immense pleasure coming from the stimulus applied to your body. When you perceive many peaks in a short period, you are getting a multiorgasm, and the ecstasy coming from it is a much more incredible feeling than whatever you'll ever sense when ejaculating.

Multiorgasm and long sexual intercourse are directly related. If you have a long and intense sensual activity, you'll get more chances to reach the multiorgasm. To achieve both results, you need to take control of your body and master your sperma release; in doing so, you'll decide the duration of your lovemaking. Don't worry. Over thousands of years, the participants in tantric sex have mastered different methods to control their ejaculation, and this section is about sharing some of those secrets.

How to last longer

The first thing to last longer is to don't ejaculate early. Ok, this is too obvious. How do you actually do that? It's pretty simple, and it's also the most difficult thing to do: don't think about ejaculating. When you are making love, you don't have to think about the grand finale; actually, you don't have to think about anything at all! In tantra is all about feeling the moment. So, clear your mind and enjoy all the pleasure coming from the experience. For this reason, relaxation is such an essential key in tantra. When you relax, your thoughts are silent, and your mind is free to enjoy any sensations coming through your body. I know. It's not very simple to don't think about ejaculating but starting with the idea to reject it is the first step for you to delay it as far as you can.

All the tantric secrets discussed until now have the purpose of reaching awareness and getting better control of your body. Therefore, all the techniques to practice tantra can help you to achieve long-sex endurance. Yoga, meditation, and pranayamas are all fundamental parts if you want to reach ejaculation-mastery. But, from all, the essential one is breath control. In tantra, you use your breath to connect with your partner. How you breathe also decides the rhythm of your lovemaking, and in tantric sex, you want to go slow. So, whenever you feel close to the peak, slow down your breath even more: try with five seconds breathing in and five seconds breathing out. If you feel comfortable, you can even try to hold your breath for a couple of seconds occasionally.

To master the control of your peak, you can also train specifically the part of your body that causes the ejaculation. I am talking about the PC muscle (or pubococcygeus muscle), situated between the pubic bone and the tail bone, forming the floor of your pelvic cavity. This muscle contracts during ejaculation and controls the urine activity too.

Now that you are aware of the existence of the PC muscle, you need to understand how to take control of it. The method is the same that you apply when you are holding your urine. To make it in practice, you can try to stop the flow while you are peeing. Next time you have to urinate, give it a try: stop the flow and then release it, stop it again and then release it, and so on. This will make you aware of the muscle that you need to train. Now that you know about this muscle, you don't have to necessary pee to improve its strength. Just contract it regularly during your everyday life, like sitting at a desk or waiting for the bus. This practice is called **Kegel exercise**, also known as **pelvic-floor exercise.**

Applying this training with regularity is a very healthy habit, not only for taking control of the ejaculation. But you need to be patient and constant with this activity because it takes about three months to see the results. Still, I promise it will be worth it! Reinforcing the pelvic floor muscle is beneficial for both women and men because it helps prevent continence and pre-ejaculation issues. Women can apply the Kegel exercise too, but I will talk about this later.

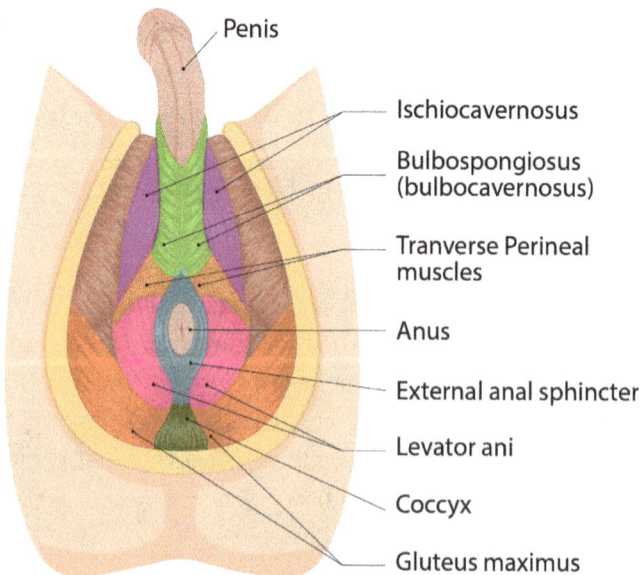

- Penis
- Ischiocavernosus
- Bulbospongiosus (bulbocavernosus)
- Tranverse Perineal muscles
- Anus
- External anal sphincter
- Levator ani
- Coccyx
- Gluteus maximus

Pompoir

There is an exciting female-centered technique in tantra where the man is slowly stimulated by the contraction of the vagina. Pompoir is a sexual technique where the woman is entirely in charge of the activity while the man is totally passive; still, he gets the best fun. This technique is also known as *kabzah*, and is also referred to as *Singapore Kiss*. The woman typically goes on the top, and she grabs and holds the partner's member contracting her vaginal muscles. The stimulation comes through muscle contraction alone, and no other actions are required, like rocking or thrusting. So, it requires much vaginal strength and contraction skills; but once the woman acquires these abilities, she will be able to provide her man one of the best sensations in his life. Training your body to apply this technique requires time and constant practice, and you need to wait from four to six months to perform it correctly. You can even use some tools to accelerate your training, like Yoni eggs or Ben wa balls, but they are in no way necessary. In the next section, I'll give you some exercises to learn how to perform pompoir for your man.

For women: practicing Pompoir

Pompoir is an action caused through the vaginal muscles to stimulate the man's member when making love with your partner. This act is meant to give pleasure to the male partner, but it's also beneficial for the woman since it gives her more empowerment during tantric sex. Having the female partner practicing with pompoir improves the sexual experience for both the subjects. Unfortunately, this practice is mainly known in Far Eastern cultures, and it arrived in the Western world just recently, especially when you come to known the tantric world.

Pompoir is not an easy skill because it's happening internally. But there are four main motions to focus on when practicing it: squeeze, contract, push and pull. But before describing these actions, let's start with the basics. I mentioned before the Kegel exercise, and I gave some instructions for the men to perform it. Now, it's time to provide some guidance for the women.

Some women may already hear about the Kegel exercises since many doctors recommend it during and after pregnancy to help prevent urinary leaking. To apply this training, you can place your finger inside your vagina and try to squeeze it with the muscles in your pelvic. Another way to practicing is to try to stop your urine mid-flow, thigh and hold for few seconds and then relax. But the last one is just a suggestion to figure out the feeling and the muscles you need to train for the pompoir. Holding your urine regularly, even for few seconds, is not a good practice for a healthy reason, so once you realized the action you need to replicate, practice with it without putting your health on the line. Once you have figured out how to squeeze your pelvic muscle, you can take any possible occasion to compress and release during your daily routine.

Once you get better with squeezing through Kegel exercises, you can try the next step: pull and push. For these actions, you need to imagine that your vagina is sucking something and than pulling it out. The movements are the same as the Kegel exercise, but you need some practice before getting it right. My suggestion is to try to understand these actions involving your partner. Next time you are busy in lovemaking, explain to your partner what you want to perform and ask him to thrust slowly. Then, with your vagina muscles, do the opposite of what he is doing: when he moves in, you push out, like if you are trying to reject him out; when he pulls out, you squeeze as you want to suck him in. This is a good training to understand how to perform it, and having your partner involved will definitely add some fun! Once you get familiar with the movements, you can practice them yourself like you are doing with the previous exercise. To perform it alone, you'll better do it on the toilet; sitting on something hollow will help you put effort into the correct muscles while the rest of the body is relaxing.

Once you acquire some skills with the pull-push, you may want to try the "twisting." As the name suggests, imagine holding a pen between the thumb and the pointer finger, and you move it from one side to the other, twisting the pen. You have to replicate the same movements with your pelvic muscles when your partner is inside you. With this type of action, not only will your man be swallowed by a wave of pleasure, but you too will enjoy his member moving around your vaginal tissue.

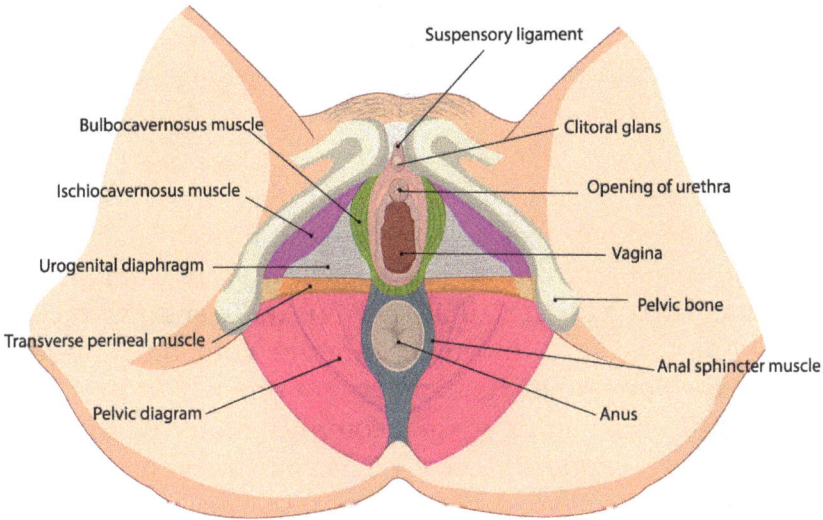

9.3 MULTIPLE ORGASMS AND LONG ORGASM

Orgasm is the final goal when having sex, and people want this experience to be excellent and unique. If having an orgasm generates the most incredible feeling of pleasure and satisfaction, having more than one in a short period can only make the experience even better. Take in mind, however, that the multiorgasm is not the final goal for tantric sex. On the contrary, people who practice Tantra aim to get one single orgasm that can last for a long time. Some veterans in tantric sex may claim to experience orgasms that may have last even half an hour.

Multiorgasm and tantric orgasm are two different experiences because however long an orgasm lasts, it's still just one orgasm.

Multiple orgasms, instead, require the first orgasm to end before starting a new one later, so there is like a break between them where the subject is relaxing a bit. Typically, the multiorgasm happens through continued or renewed stimulation.

Saying if the multiorgasm experience is worst or better than a long-period orgasm is entirely subjective. Some people may prefer one or the other depending on their idea of great pleasure. Either way, both the experiences are worth trying, and tantric sex can help make them happen. Following some guidelines to help you with them.

Keep your cool

This may sound unusual, yet the best way by which you can defer your intercourse is by keeping your cool. On the off chance that you feel that your peak is snappy moving closer, you have to calm down, limiting your breathing and pushing developments. Remember that one key to tantric sex is communication, so let your accomplice know why you are slowing down, even if the best is for you two to agree on the same goals before starting the intercourse.

Go gradually

When you start participating in tantric sex with your accomplice, guarantee that you are taking things progressively. The more slow the sex is, the more outstanding your peak would be, an immediate consequence of all the turn of events.

Calm yourself, obstruct your breathing, and handle your pelvic muscles.

When you feel that your peak is subsiding, relax a bit and calm down your breath; after a short time, you can eventually proceed with your pushing development. Keep repeating this methodology for whatever time that you can hold off. Develop your energy and keep going. This advancement will make your peak last more, and it will be even more noteworthy. When you feel that you are close to peak, endeavor and grasp your pubic muscles while still going on. It will not simply hold you back from releasing; it will also allow you to encounter the joy of a peak and not lose your erection, which means that you will be able to prop up extensively in the wake of experiencing an orgasm. After some practice, you will have the alternative to hold off for quite a while longer and participate in sexual relations for a significant long time together.

Conclusion

When you learn about tantric sex, you realize how the perception built around the act of love is a matter of mindset. Some people feel guilty when talking about sex and prefer to keep all their naughty experiences locked away. Others may talk about sex shamelessly and feel proud of their achievements and performances. Sex in modern life is a topic full of contradictions and challenges. It's described as one of the most beautiful experiences in life, but at the same time, it is considered a perverted and sinful act.

Considering these contradictions, it's pretty clear why some couples feel reluctant to talk about sex, sometimes even between each other. Whatever you are facing troubles in your relationship or looking for new tips and emotions to bring into your sexual activity, finding the right person and moment to ask for advice can be challenging.

This is where Tantra can come as an answer for some couples facing this dilemma. Tantra is a journey that opens our minds and can help us to live with harmony and accept divinity in our lives. It teaches how to find balance, accept pleasure and feelings as they come, and make use of them to contemplate the beauty of the material and spiritual world. Although most people associate Tantra only with sex, it's a much deeper discipline. Following, I want to summarize some of the teachings I learned along my journey, hoping that they can come in handy for you while finding your own path.

It's not only about sex

Associate tantra automatically to sex is a misconception. Tantra is not about prolonged and uncontrolled sexual intercourse, as assumed by many. Sex is a primary instinct instilled in human nature to ensure the species survive. Tantra has a much deeper meaning; it does make use of sexual energy in a constructive way. Through Tantra, we want to explore our limitations and overcome them.

For this reason, Tantra is neither a religion nor a science but a spiritual journey. It's an instrument that allows the individual to deeper understand themselves and improve through the development of mind and body. The objective of Tantra is to have the option to work with your accomplice together to accomplish an absolute pleasure and cause the other individual to feel better. In any case, you don't need orgasm as the objective. Instead, you should cooperate to make yourself both upbeat and fulfilled.

It's about knowing your body

Like yoga, tantra is all about physical and spiritual awareness. When you walk the path of tantra, you take more consciousness about your body and your areas of pleasure. There is nothing to be ashamed about; you need to consider yourself as a divinity, and your body is the temple that brings you to heaven. Remember that the word "tantra" means "to wave" because everything is connected, as your body is connected to your internal energy that flows in powerful waves. Knowing yourself is the first step to get in contact with your spirit and the entire Universe.

It's about knowing your partner

In most cases, when a couple approaches Tantra is to add some fun into their relationship. Indeed, Tantra may sound exciting and inspiring, but it's also a discipline that requires seriousness and devotion. When you apply tantric teachings with your partner, you start a spiritual journey together, which can bring the two of you to a profound bond. Using Tantra in a relationship means to be physically aware and spiritually present for each other. You approve to exchange your energies with one another, keeping this connection even after the orgasm. Staring this journey together will allow you to understand each other better. This is not only about discovering the erogenous zones of your partner's body but exploring their soul.

You Might not Get it Right the First Time

Most people approach Tantra to have better and longer sex, and they expect to get results in short times. But there are no such things as short-cuts in life, and Tantra is no exception. So, whatever is the reason that brings you close to this philosophy, you will have to try multiple times before seeing any results. You may search for the best sex in your life, or maybe you are just willing to bring some fun into your relationship, but if you don't practice, you'll never get whatever you want to achieve. It's a sort of training that requires persistence, and you should consistently put aside the time you go through with your partner. So, don't get frustrated if you won't see any changes the first time you are doing tantric sex. Don't give up at the beginning, and you'll get there one step per time.

Take it slow and enjoy the trip

We are so busy with everyday life that we don't have time to relax and enjoy the beauty in the world. With sex, the problem is similar. We rush so much to reach the orgasm, and in the end, we'll end up with bitter and incomplete satisfaction. Tantra teaches the opposite. To take things slow, to enjoy the moment, and to relax instead of rushing. This teaching is applied for Tantra in sex as in life. Too often, we live in expectations, and we are too busy aiming the target that we are blind to everything else. It's good to set up goals because they lead us to what we want, and they give us the time to organize. Even for tantric sex, it's a good practice to have it planned with your partner to have everything ready in time. But starting with a goal in mind doesn't necessarily mean ignoring whatever is not on your path. Sometimes it's nice to step back and enjoy the journey.

I am aware that Tantra is a very profound discipline and this book scratches only the surface of the topic. My purpose was to give you some basic knowledge about this fascinating culture without neglecting the fun that comes with it. I did my best to cover both theory and practice to provide you with a general understanding and getting you in touch with the basics. Now it's up to you to decide to go deep with this path and apply it regularly in your everyday life or use the knowledge provided for occasional fun. Either way, I hope this book will guide you along your journey and contribute to improving your life.